Evaluation and Management of Allergic and Asthmatic Diseases

Evaluation and Management of Allergic and Asthmatic Diseases

Edited by

M. Eric Gershwin, M.D., F.A.C.P.

and

Stephen M. Nagy, Jr., M.D.

Section of Rheumatology-Allergy
Department of Medicine
University of California
Davis, California

GRUNE & STRATTON
A Subsidiary of Harcourt Brace Jovanovich, Publishers
New York   San Francisco   London

Grune & Stratton, Inc.
111 Fifth Avenue
New York, New York 10003

Distributed in the United Kingdom by
Academic Press, Inc. (London) Ltd.
24/28 Oval Road, London NW 1

Library of Congress Catalog Number 79-1987
International Standard Book Number 0-8089-1206-2
Printed in the United States of America

Contents

Objectives and Introduction

To many physicians, allergy represents a discipline only slightly less sterile than a Johnson & Johnson gauze pad, a pursuit followed by dilettanti, pseudoscholastic beatniks, and eccentric professors. To others, it is only a subsection of modified acupuncture. Yet allergic phenomena, like respiration and digestion, are ubiquitous functions of man in nature and remain key and critical sources of morbidity. The social and family strains, the economic stress, and the personal anguish all rival or exceed other chronic diseases. Yet few physicians are prepared to do more than commiserate for the pathos and misery involved. Fortunately, this dismal picture shows signs of impending remission. The disciplines of clinical immunology and allergy have made enormous strides in the past decade—probably more so than any branch of medicine and physiology (sic, it had the longest to go). Newer clinics and more sophisticated pharmacology of these agents are available. In this volume, it is our objective to impart many of these concepts to the practicing physician. Our success depends heavily on the use of clinical/applied material; theoretical basic science will be used only in terms of relevant physiology. It is our hope that this approach, including the self-assessment examination, will be individually useful and productive.

We would like to express our appreciation to the many people who helped in the organization of this book. First, our thanks to Dr. Neil Andrews, Helen Miller, Nancy Kluth and Pam McNally of the Department of Post-Graduate Medicine, from which the nucleus of our thoughts arose; second, thanks to Leona Schmidt and Deborah Ackerman for their careful secretarial input, and finally, to Richard Beach, David Eckels, Richard Menning and John Montero for their proofreading.

Contributors

JAMES J. CASTLES, M.D.
Section of Rheumatology-Allergy
Department of Medicine
University of California
Davis, California

PAUL CLONINGER, M.D.
Section of Rheumatology-Allergy
Department of Medicine
University of California
Davis, California

PAUL J. DONALD, M.D.
Department of Otorhinolaryngology
University of California
Davis, California

RALPH C. FRATES, JR., M.D.
Department of Pediatrics
University of California
Davis, California

M. ERIC GERSHWIN, M.D., F.A.C.P.
Section of Rheumatology-Allergy
Department of Medicine
University of California
Davis, California

MICHAEL H. KESLIN, M.D.
Section of Rheumatology-Allergy
Department of Medicine
University of California
Davis, California

MICHAEL A. KLASS, M.D.
Department of Dermatology
University of California
Davis, California

GLEN A. LILLINGTON, M.D., F.R.C.P. (C), F.A.C.P.
Section of Pulmonary Medicine
Department of Medicine
University of California
Davis, California

STANLEY M. NAGUWA, M.D.
Section of Rheumatology-Allergy
Department of Medicine
University of California
Davis, California

STEPHEN M. NAGY, JR., M.D.
Section of Rheumatology-Allergy
Department of Medicine
University of California
Davis, California

HAROLD S. NOVEY, M.D.
Section of Allergy
Department of Medicine
University of California
Irvine, California

STEPHEN R. STEWART, M.D.
Section of Rheumatology-Allergy
Department of Medicine
University of California
Davis, California

MARTIN D. VALENTINE, M.D.
Department of Allergy
Johns Hopkins School of Medicine
Baltimore, Maryland

JOSEPH M. YOUNG, M.D.
Section of Rheumatology-Allergy
Department of Medicine
University of California
Davis, California

Evaluation and Management of Allergic and Asthmatic Diseases

Stephen M. Nagy, Jr.

THE ALLERGIC HISTORY

INTRODUCTION

In my first clinical lecture as a second year medical
student, it was confidently stated that the history
would provide the diagnosis in 85% of patients. How
such a figure was derived is anyone's guess and presumably it originated as merely a rough estimate. Indeed,
no one thought to challenge our faculty in those days.
Today, however, some bright young person would certainly
ask for the reference, perhaps in ungrammatical fashion.
Indeed, although the last two decades have been marked
by an incredible explosion of biomedical information,
there has certainly not been a concurrent increase in
verbal skills. One has only to listen to current con-
versations so frequently punctuated by "you knows," to
understand the depths of the problem. "You know" is a
euphemism which, roughly translated, means "you know
what I mean, at least I hope you do, since I don't have
the skill to express myself." The art (or science) of
history taking has suffered along much the same lines.
In allergy, common "you know" phrases include "hay fever
symptoms," "allergy-type symptoms," "itchy rash" and
"chest problems." It is impressionism come to medicine,
but unlike the visual art, lacks specificity, quantitation, and even a theoretical rationale. The relegation
of the history to the completion of a form, a computer,
or to non-medical office personnel reflects another example of its declining place in our diagnostic armamentarium. Part of this disdain is understandable. The
laboratory has usurped the diagnostician as the final
authority in various disease entities and it, therefore,
may seem fruitless to list a host of symptoms in a
jaundiced patient.
This attitude takes a narrow view for it presumes

3

the <u>sole</u> function of the history is to catalog pertinent
social, genealogical and medical facts, as well as
current symptoms. *Materia medica* are only incidental to
the crucial initial portion of an interview where one
evaluates communication skills, reliability and memory.
Medical jargon is not the language of the outsider.
Does the patient distinguish pain from discomfort or
fullness, itching from burning, congestion from sputa,
wheezing from snoring, or rash from itching (pruritus)?
Are the usual landmarks, i.e. residences, marriages,
operations, serious illnesses, accurately recalled?
Are past diagnoses properly chronicled or riddled with
internal inconsistencies such as "I had a heart attack",
but was hospitalized for only two days, "I had pneumonia seven times last year" without chest films being
obtained, or "I don't take aspirin", but "Alka-Seltzer"
is used regularly. Words should be sifted, phrases
weighed; the process is intensely analytical, a veiled
inquisition, not an informal chat.

Traditionally, the interview is divided into five
areas, social history, family history, past medical
history, present illness, and review of systems.
Figures 1 and 2 display a history form for use by the
physician on which the following discussion is based.
It not only organizes and outlines pertinent facts,
especially areas not customarily explored, it also
allows for the rapid retrieval of specific points of
information when evaluating subsequent problems.
Further, it can readily be adapted to problem-oriented
record approaches. It is meant as a guide particularly
for physicians unfamiliar with the critical answers and
information required for allergic evaluations. Indeed,
to return to the issue of information gathering above,
the history in allergy evaluations remains an overwhelming help to the diagnostician.

SOCIAL HISTORY

Allergy histories in the great majority deal in con-
stellations of nasal and/or pulmonary symptoms. In
order to properly evaluate the chronology of these
symptoms, and especially to be able to relate them to
specific exposures, it is important to know where the

patient has resided and for what periods of time. Even
moves within a state, and to a lesser extent within a
city, may result in significant changes in environmental
flora. At times, even the new residence may have been
an unbeknownst repository of a menangerie. Animal ped-
igree and exposure should be carefully documented.
Small, frequently shampooed poodles seldom produce the
problems of a German shepard with the run of the house.
Siamese cats are seldom outdoors in spite of protesta-
tions to the contrary. Other households with primarily
indoor pets are frequently consciously avoided. Childhood attachments or recent changes in bedding, i.e.
pillows, blankets, comforters, elucidate a chronic exposure to feathers, wool or down. Occupational exposures are so important that a chapter (p. 113) of this
volume has been devoted to this topic.

The deleterious effects of cigarette smoking on nasal
and bronchial membranes require little emphasis. More
recent studies, however, indicate that even asthmatic
children of smoking parents present to emergency rooms
more frequently than those of non-smokers.

Alcohol use, even in moderate amounts reduces ciliary
function and, therefore, adversely effects pulmonary
clearance mechanisms. In large amounts, chronic aspiration becomes more likely. The social implications
need little discussion.

FAMILY HISTORY

In important clinical studies, all progeny are evaluated directly. Genealogical histories are almost
always obtained second-hand, unless the entire family
is under one's care. The point is that they are of
limited value. Is mother's chronic rash eczema or
psoriasis? Is grandfather's wheezing secondary to
asthma or chronic bronchitis? Are brother's sinus complaints infectious or allergic in etiology? Skillful
probing may produce a pretty accurate guess, but this
depends on a thorough knowledge of the atopic diseases,
their course, variant aspects, and therapy. And, in
spite of their familial tendency, it is still incumbent
upon the practitioner to establish the diagnosis in the
patient. I have usually found such histories more

helpful when they are void of atopic problems and, therefore, support a non-atopic diagnosis. One important exception is food allergy and, if positive, may rapidly lead to appropriate diets and a grateful patient Finally, the only clues, besides the illness itself, to the classically inherited "non-allergic" diseases, cystic fibrosis and hereditary angio-edema, may reside here.

PAST MEDICAL HISTORY

This outlines important medical landmarks, i.e. operations, hospitalizations, injuries and serious illnesses that may not have or currently do not require in-hospital treatment. Specifically, tonsil, adenoid, nasal and sinus surgery and the indications thereof should be completely explored. Repeated respiratory exacerbations, especially requiring hospitalization, should be documented as to season if not month. Such diagnoses as "pulmonary emboli," "cardiac failure," "coronary insufficiency," or "an infectious illness," all of which have common symptomatology, require substantiation by both history and even requisition of appropriate records.

Hypertension, coronary artery disease, valvular disease, arrhythmias, and the arthridides lead to the use of certain drugs, i.e. propanolol, reserpine, aspirin and other anti-inflammatory compounds, which create de novo or exacerbate asthmatic and nasal syndromes. Phenothiazines, commonly utilized in neurotic and psychotic disorders, produce mild to moderate nasal dryness and congestion. In fact, new patients should be encouraged to bring in a list of all medications, i.e. antacids, cold remedies, hormones, analgesics, taken in the previous year. They also provide clues to illnesses poorly understood or simply forgotten.

An important subsection within the past medical history undertakes to discuss prior events or illnesses that may have had an immunological basis. Primary in this category are reactions to drugs. Once the medication and route of administration are identified, the history should attempt to differentiate the classical types of reactions, i.e. overdosage, intolerance, idiosyncrasy, side or secondary effect from the allergic

reaction. No part of the history is probably more de-
linquent than this in accepting a patient's diagnosis
without proper substantiation.

Urticarial episodes, their severity, duration, distribution and possible etiology should be documented.
For a more complete discussion of the significance of
these episodes, see page 189-204. Reactions to stinging and/or biting insects should be explored both as to
the identification of the insect and the severity of
the reaction. (See page 247).

Food sensitivities and intolerances are extensively
reviewed in a separate chapter. Although infant feeding problems are related "second hand," they are
usually worth pursuing as they may persist into adult
life in a more mild form. Colic, repeated episodes
of vomiting, chronic nasal congestion, and intermittent
diarrhea represent the spectrum of milk intolerance.
Dietary modifications, their effectiveness and the subsequent reintroduction of milk should all be recorded.
Intertwined with this may be a history of atopic dermatitis and its distribution, duration, seasonal
changes, therapy and associations with diet should also
be explored.

Adults are more likely to suffer from recurrent gastrointestinal complaints, specifically excessive flatus,
cramps or diarrhea with specific foods. A diagnosis of
or treatment for chronic colonic complaints even in the
absence of associations with specific foods, should
be recorded here or in the past medical history. Relationships of foods to nasal or asthmatic symptoms
are usually explored in the present illness. Lastly,
approximately six percent of patients with pollenosis
complain of an oral pruritus with melons and/or banana
and/or avocados. This ranges from a sensation of itching
of the palate and pharynx to actual swelling and mild
laryngeal symptoms. Chronic otitis, particularly in
childhood is frequently related either to chronic inhalant sensitivity or milk sensitivity or intolerance
and its duration and treatment should be recorded.

PRESENT ILLNESS

Although a few questions are expended at the very

outset of the interview to determine the patient's
major complaints, the major discussion of these symptoms
should be left to its final portion. Each aspect of
the history is important, but this is certainly the
most crucial and for years it has behooved me to understand why medical schools persist in teaching their
students to begin there. Just as a painter's first task
is composition, followed by landscape and finally the
major figures, so the narrative of nasal, pulmonary,
skin or gastrointestinal symptoms should unfold with
the perspective of social, genealogical and past medical relationships. Symptoms may then be plotted graph-
ically against exposures, drugs, travel, stress and
other factors that relate to alterations of environ-
ments.

The initial task is an exact definition of complaints. As outlined previously, allergic histories
deal mainly in nasal and pulmonary symptoms, less frequently with skin problems, i.e. atopic dermatitis and
urticaria, and only occasionally with drug reactions
and gastrointestinal complaints. The symptoms referable
to each area should be examined specifically and outlined chronologically. Does "congestion" mean nasal
obstruction, sinus pressure, chest tightness or wheezing? Is the appropriate translation of the initial
complaint, "right sinus fullness," more correctly a
throbbing right sided headache? Once defined, they
undergo retrospective analysis. Has there been a progression, i.e. throat clearing to cough to chest tightness to frank wheezing or are they stable with mild
occasional exacerbations? Figure 1 outlines a schematic to plot seasonal changes as well as a check list
of common exacerbating factors which should be assigned
values based on individual sensitivity. Severity is,
of course, arbitrary. A more accurate index may reside
in more substantial and defineable landmarks such as
frequency of office visits, emergency room visits, hospitalizations, missed school or work disability. The
patient's requirement for and response to various medications may be even a more objective assessment.
Asthma adequately treated with "Benadryl," is clearly
not as critical as that requiring steroids. Unrespon-
siveness of classical seasonal nasal and eye symptoms
to over the counter antihistamine decongestants is a

FIGURE 1

HISTORY

SH-birthplace   residences

  marital status

  occupation(s)

  military service

  tobacco

  EtOH

  pets

  Other

FH-mother

  father

  siblings

  children

      diabetes, tbc, hypertension, heart disease,
      arthritis, Ca, asthma, hayfever, eczema, other:

      food allergies

PH-Operations

  Hospitalizations

Illnesses

Injuries

Medications

  allergy   other:

  Vits

  ASA

  hormones

Past Allergic History-drug reactions

                    urticaria

                    food sensitivities

                    insect stings

                    asthma

                    hayfever

                    eczema

                    otitis

Present Illness

Exacerbating Factors-   Nasal   Pulmonary

        travel

        exercise

        change in temp.

        dust

        animals

        foods

        infection

        stress

        drugs (ASA)

        outside

        irritants

        smoke

Seasonal	Jan	Feb	Mar	Apr	May	June	July	Aug	Sept	Oct
Nasal										
Pulmonary										

Seasonal	Nov	Dec
Nasal		
Pulmonary		

Response to Medications-Nasal Sxs

                Pulmonary Sxs

System Review

crucial feature, not only in assessing severity, but in
determining further evaluation and therapy. Prior
allergic management, i.e. skin testing and hyposensitization bespeaks of more than trivial problems.

   This chapter cannot cover every symptom and every disease process. The remainder of this volume, however
attempts to give the physician more perspective on the
signs and symptoms of classical "allergic" disorders,
their evaluation and management. In so doing, it as-
pires to make the preceding a more knowledgeable and
fruitful process. Moreover it fosters a warm physician-
patient relationship; something that is very critical
in the long term management of allergic patients.

REFERENCES

Coca, AF, Cooke, RA: On the classification of the phenomena of hypersensitiveness. J. Immunol. 8:163,1923.
Roitt, I: Essential immunology, ed. 2,Oxford, England,
   1974, Blackwell Scientific Publications.
Farr, RS, Spector, SL: What is asthma? In Petty, TL,
   editor: The asthmatic patient in trouble, Greenwich,
   Conn., 1975, C.P.C. Communications, Inc.

Stanley Naguwa
and James J. Castles

MEDIATORS OF THE ALLERGIC INFLAMMATORY RESPONSE

INTRODUCTION

The allergic inflammatory response has both bio-chemical and cellular components. This chapter will discuss the biochemical mediators. The bulk of the data on biochemical mediators are from animal studies. However, because of interspecies response differences, the data from studies of human tissue will be emphasized.

HYPOTHETICAL CASE

A 20 year old college student is brought to the Emergency Room of the hospital in respiratory distress and vascular collapse. History provided by friends who have brought him reveals that he had just returned from the student clinic after being treated for a presumed strep throat before suddenly becoming ill. On physical examination, the vital signs are blood pressure 80/50, pulse 100 and thready, and respiratory rate 24 and labored. Wheezing is heard on auscultation of the chest. Immediate resuscitation is begun with intrave-nous fluids and epinephrine. Aminophylline is then started after a loading dose. Slowly the student im-proves and is able to give a prior history of allergic rhinitis with sore throats occasionally treated with penicillin.

The preceding case illustrates several important features of an anaphylactic reaction to penicillin. First, there was prior exposure to the offending anti-gen, the sine qua non of anaphylaxis. Second, the reac-tion was immediate. Third, vascular collapse and bronchospasm are the prominent and life threatening components of the anaphylactic reaction. Last, correct initial treatment was given with fluids and epinephrine.

Histamine, slow-reacting substance of anaphylaxis
(SRS-A), eosinophilic chemotactic factor of anaphylaxis
(ECF-A), basophilic kallikrein of anaphylaxis (BK-A),
and platelet activating factor (PAF) are released by
sensitized tissue after IgE-antigen interaction. As
they are released directly as a result of the reaginic
reaction, they are termed primary mediators. In contrast, serotonin, bradykinin, and prostaglandins are
released in response to the primary mediators or to the
allergic inflammatory reaction in general. An important factor to emphasize is that these mediators are
released concurrently or sequentially and work in
concert to produce the allergic inflammatory response.

VASCULAR CHANGES

The vascular changes in the allergic inflammatory
response may be systemic or localized.

Anaphylaxis

Systemic: generalized urticaria,
angioedema, vascular
collapse.

Localized: urticaria, localized
angioedema.

However, the mediators that cause these effects are
identical, with the best understood of them being
histamine.

HISTAMINE

Histamine was the first mediator of the allergic
inflammatory response identified and of which the most
is known. The foundation for understanding its role
was laid down by the work of Dale and Laidlaw in 1910
and 1919. They correctly noted that histamine, while
playing a significant role in anaphylaxis, was not the
sole mediator. Histamine, or 5-beta-imidazolylethyla-
mine, is a low molecular weight amine formed primarily
by the decarboxylation of L-histidine in human mast
cells, basophils, gastrointestinal tract, and central
nervous system. It is stored in intracellular granules as a histamine mucopolysaccharide complex. The

mast cells have the highest content per unit weight of
tissue and represent the most important individual cell
in the allergic inflammatory response. Basophils also
are important in the anaphylactic response, whereas the
histamine in the gastrointestinal tract and central
nervous system is thought to act as a local mediator not
associated with anaphylaxis.

Histamine release has been studied using fragments
of human sensitized lung tissue and leukocytes with pur-
ified antigen in strictly controlled conditions. Release
is a noncytotoxic, energy dependent, calcium requiring
process, and is modulated by changes in the intracellular levels of cyclic AMP and cyclic GMP by catechola-
mines (which induce adenyl cyclase), cholinergic stimulation (which increase guanidyl cyclase), histamine
itself by desensitization of a mast cell, and prostaglandins (which alter cyclic AMP or cyclic GMP, depending on specific type).

Figure 1.

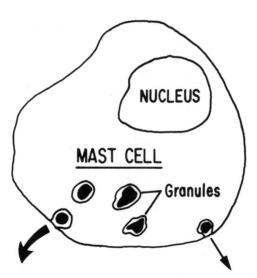

Increased Release (inc cAMP)   Decreased released (inc cGMP)

β-adrenergic stimulation   Cholinergic stimulation
Pg F   Pg F
Phosphodiesterase inhibitors   Histamine
C3a, C5a

Work with antihistamines has shown that both the
H_1 and H_2 receptors cause vasodilation and increased
vascular permeability. The latter results from the
separation of venular endothelial cells. Locally these
changes cause urticaria, when superficial, and angio-
edema when the deeper layers of connective tissue are
involved. If the vascular effects are pronounced, the
"effective" intravascular volume may be depleted to the
point of hypotension.

SLOW-REACTING SUBSTANCE OF ANAPHYLAXIS (SRS-A)

Since antihistamines do not block all the events
in the anaphylactic reaction, particularly that of
bronchospasm, other mediators were searched for and a
low molecular weight acidic sulfur-containing substance
was identified. Yet to be well characterized, it was
named slow-reacting substance of anaphylaxis (SRS-A),
as tests with guinea pig ileum, the standard assay for
smooth muscle contraction, demonstrated that the substance produced a slower rate of contraction than
histamine. Kinetic studies have shown that SRS-A is
not pre-formed but is rapidly synthesized by mast cells
after IgE-antigen interaction. Maximum intracellular
levels are reached in two minutes and extracellular in
two to thirty minutes in tests using human lung
fragments. Formation and release of SRS-A are dependent upon antigen concentration and the response is
modulated by cyclic nucleotides as with histamine (see
Figure 1). In addition to causing bronchospasm, SRS-A
also increases vascular permeability and thus enhances
the effects of histamine.

BASOPHILS

Studies of the basophil revealed still another
mediator, basophilic kallikrein of anaphylaxis or BK-A,
which is pre-formed and found in basophils and mast
cells. BK-A has an arginine esterase activity which
activates the kinin system during anaphylaxis by cleav-
ing kininogen to release bradykinin which then causes
vasodilatation and increased vascular permeability. The
amount of BK-A released is dependent on antigen concentration and it also is modulated by cyclic nucleotides.

Basophils also release an 1100 molecular weight substance which causes specific aggregation and degranulation of platelets. This substance has been named platelet activating factor (PAF) and is responsible for the release of 5-hydroxytryptamine (5-HT), or serotonin, that the platelets have absorbed and stored in intracellular granules. Serotonin increases vascular permeability.

BRONCHOSPASM

Like the vascular changes, several mediators work in concert to produce the bronchospasm seen in anaphylaxis. Bronchial smooth muscle contraction is caused by histamine, SRS-A, bradykinin, complement fragments, and serotonin. The serotonin effect is weak compared to histamine. Because of the number of mediators that can cause bronchospasm, the use of antagonists to treat this feature is less than optimal, and direct acting bronchodilators acutely are generally required.

MODULATION OF THE ALLERGIC INFLAMMATORY REACTION

The biochemical mediators also serve to modulate the allergic inflammatory response. Histamine itself has a direct negative feedback effect on the mast cell inhibiting further release of this substance. At histamine concentrations that saturate the H_1 receptors, H_2 receptors are activated which cause a decrease in lymphocyte effector functions, decreased PMN chemotaxis, and increased chemotaxis of eosinophils. The latter role is shared with eosinophilic chemotactic factor (ECF-A) which is a group of peptides found pre-formed in mast cells and released upon reaginic stimulation. Eosinophils have enzymes which metabolize the biochemical mediators, thereby limiting the anaphylactic reaction. Serotonin works in concert with the other substances by decreasing lymphocyte mediator release.

PROSTAGLANDINS

Prostaglandins are discussed separately because the precise role that they play in the anaphylactic reaction is not known. Prostaglandins are a ubiquitous

group of related substances that are pre-formed in almost all tissues and possibly rapidly synthesized from
cell wall breakdown products during the inflammatory
response. Prostaglandins are also released from eosinophils upon reaginic stimulation.

    The following is a summary of prostaglandin
effects:

	Effect on cyclic nucleotides	Direct effect
Prostaglandin E	Increase c-AMP	Increase vascular permeability.
Prostaglandin F	Increase c-GMP	Increase vascular permeability, weak.
Thromboxane		Smooth muscle contraction.

    Relative levels or balance of the cyclic nucleotide
levels will determine the enhancement (cyclic AMP) or
inhibition (cyclic GMP) of histamine release. This may
be an important factor or partial explanation of the
dichotomy of effects on asthmatic patients by the prostaglandin synthetase inhibitors, e.g. acetylsalicylic
acid, indomethacin.

COMPLEMENT SYSTEM

    It is unknown whether or not the complement system
plays a significant role in anaphylaxis. However, vasoactive proteins are released during complement system
activation and may have a role in the anaphylactic
reaction. The following is a schematic of the complement activation sequence.

```
      C1        C4        C2        C3        C5
Ag-Ab──Ag AbC1──AgAbC14──AgAbC142──AgAbC1423──AgAbC14235
                         │          │           │
                      C-kinin      C3a         C5a
```

C-kinin has "bradykinin-like" effects but differs
chemically. Both C3a and C5a have direct vascular per-

meability effects and also can stimulate histamine release.

ANAPHYLACTOID REACTIONS

Most anaphylactic reactions result from an IgE-Ag interaction which directly causes the release of the biochemical mediators. On the other hand, morphine, polymyxin B, iodinated contrast agents, dextran, trauma, burns, and infection can directly cause the release of histamine which can resemble the anaphylactic reaction.

SUMMARY

The following table briefly summarizes the biochemical mediators:

Mediator	Composition	Pre-formed or Synthesized	1° Actions
Histamine	5-β-imidazo-lylethylamine	Pre-formed	Increase vascular permeability, bronchospasm.
SRS-A	Acidic sulfate ester	Synthesized	Increase vascular permeability, bronchospasm.
BK-A	?	Pre-formed	Cleaves kininogen to release bradykinin.
PAF	?	Synthesized	Aggregation and degranulation of platelets.

(to be continued)

Mediator	Composition	Pre-formed or Synthesized	1° Actions
Bradykinin	Arg-pro-pro-gly-phe-ser-pro-phe-arg	Cleaved from kininogen.	Increase vascular permeability, bronchospasm.
Serotonin	5-hydroxytryptamine	Pre-formed	Increase vascular permeability, bronchospasm.
ECF-A	Tetrapeptides: Val-gly-ser-glu Ala-gly-ser-glu	Pre-formed, synthesized	Chemotaxis of eosinophils.
Complement fragments		Released during complement system activation.	Increased vascular permeability. Chemtaxis of PMN
Prostaglandins	Fatty acids	? Pre-formed ? Synthesized	Increase vascular permeability, bronchospasm, affects mediator release, chemotaxis.

REFERENCES

Austen KF: Systemic anaphylaxis in the human being.
    NEJM 291: 661-664, 1974.
Lewis RA, Goetzl EJ, Wasserman SI, et al.: The release
    of four mediators of immediate hypersensitivity
    from human leukemic basophils. J Immunol 114:
    87-92, 1975.

Plaut M, Lichtenstein LM: Cellular and chemical basis
    of the allergic inflammatory response.   IN:
    Allergy Principles and Practice, Middleton E,
    Reed CE, Ellis EF (eds.).   The C.V. Mosby Co.
    St. Louis, Mo., 1978.
Rocha e Silva M, Garcia Leme J.:   Chemical Mediators of
    the Acute Inflammatory Reaction.   Permagon Press.
    New York, NY, 1972.
Weissman G (ed.):   Mediators of Inflammation.   Plenum
    Press.   New York, NY, 1974.

Stanley M. Naguwa

CLINICAL OBSERVATIONS OF POLLINOSIS

INTRODUCTION

A knowledge of the flora in a particular locale is important in the management of pollinosis. A physician who has first-hand knowledge of the local flora and their pollinating season can reasonably select an accurate etiologic diagnosis and thus choose the appropriate antigen for hyposensitization therapy. For example, January pollinosis in Sacramento will be due to tree pollen, specifically acacia and alder, and NOT grasses which pollinate later in the year. Though a patient may show skin test positivity to Timothy grass and Eastern ragweed, inclusion of these antigens in a hyposensitization therapy mixture while in California, for example, would not be appropriate, as these plants are absent here.

BOTANICAL OBSERVATIONS

A basic knowledge of botany is useful in the understanding of pollinosis. It is the pollen, dispersed from the anther of the flower that concerns allergists. The flower may be perfect, that is, possessing both male (stamen) and female (pistil) components (Figure 1). An example is the flower of the olive tree. Other plants, such as the Russian thistle, may have separate male and female flowers on the same plant. Lastly, there are plants that bear only one type of flower. For a patient with pollinosis, this would be helpful to know when planting a cottonwood or willow tree, during landscaping, as only the male tree would be antigenic. Though plants such as Lamb's Quarter and Mexican Tea appear grossly different in the field, they belong to the same genus—Chenopodium (sp. album - Lamb's Quarter, ambrosioides - Mexican Tea)—and are similar microscopically. It is our impression that certain plants

23

belonging to the same genus have cross-reacting antigens, e.g. Lamb's Quarter - Mexican Tea, Aspen - Cottonwood.

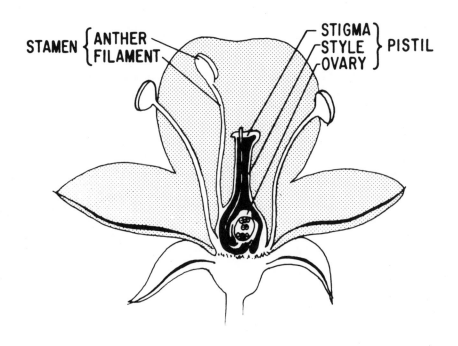

Others, such as olive - ash (olive family) and alder -
birch (birch family) do not cross-react.

HOW DO I SUSPECT WHETHER A PLANT IS ALLERGENIC?

There are criteria that one can use as a guide:

1. They must be abundant.

2. The pollens must be wind-borne and must be read-

ily found in the air. Devices such as the intermittent rotoslide are used for this purpose.

3. The flowers tend to be inconspicuous.

4. Pollen size tends to be small, about 20 microns,
in general.

5. There should be a positive clinical correlation
between symptoms and exposure to the plant.

6. The patient should demonstrate the presence of
specific IgE against the allergen in question.

POLLINATION IN TIME AND LOCATION

In general, trees tend to pollinate from January to
April. Olive tree pollinates in May, and some elm
trees pollinate even in the fall. April and May are,
generally, the peak of the grass season (in California)
with minor variations depending on the rainfall. There
are also grasses that pollinate all year 'round, such
as Bermuda grass and ryegrass. In areas such as Ha-
waii, where rainfall is perennial, grass pollen allergy
can present at any time. The weed season ranges from
August to October, or until the rain or snow arrives.
Areas such as the mountains, oceanside, or desert tend
to have much lower pollen concentration, and pollen
sensitive patients will frequently give a history of
alleviation of symptoms in these areas.

GEOGRAPHIC CONDITIONS

Climatic conditions and geography are major factors
in plant growth; this will be discussed as it relates
to pollenosis. The Northeast U.S. generally has a temperate climate and moderate rainfall which supports
abundant plant growth which is modified, however, by
the urban centers along the coast. Thus both cultivated grasses, shrubs and trees and native varieties are
important in pollinosis. The landform slowly rises
from the coast to the Appalachian mountains with native hardwood forests at the higher elevations and
grasses and cultivated trees found close to the popu-

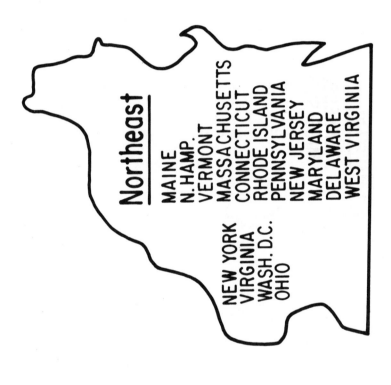

Northeast

MAINE
N.HAMP.
VERMONT
MASSACHUSETTS
CONNECTICUT
RHODE ISLAND
PENNSYLVANIA
NEW JERSEY
MARYLAND
DELAWARE
WEST VIRGINIA
NEW YORK
VIRGINIA
WASH. D.C.
OHIO

Trees: Ash, Birch, Cottonwood, Elder, Elm, Hickory
Grasses: Orchard grass, Poa spp., Redtop, Timothy
Weeds: Amaranthus spp., Cocklebur, Lamb's Quarter, Plantain, Ragweed, Rumex spp.

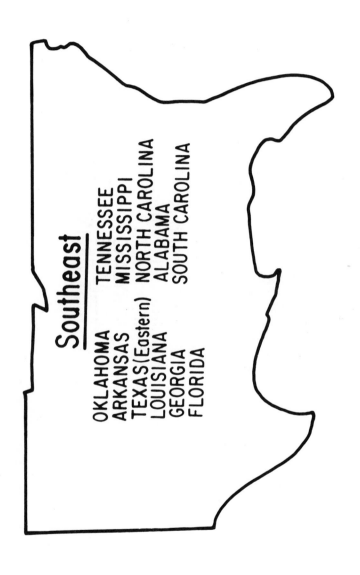

Southeast

OKLAHOMA   TENNESSEE
ARKANSAS   MISSISSIPPI
TEXAS (Eastern)   NORTH CAROLINA
LOUISIANA   ALABAMA
GEORGIA   SOUTH CAROLINA
FLORIDA

Trees: Ash, Cedar, Cottonwood, Elder, Elm, Oak
Grasses: Bermuda grass, Johnson grass, Orchard grass, Poa spp., Redtop, Rye, Timothy
Weeds: Amaranthus spp., Cocklebur, Lamb's Quarter, Plantain, Ragweed, Rumex spp.,
          Sage

28

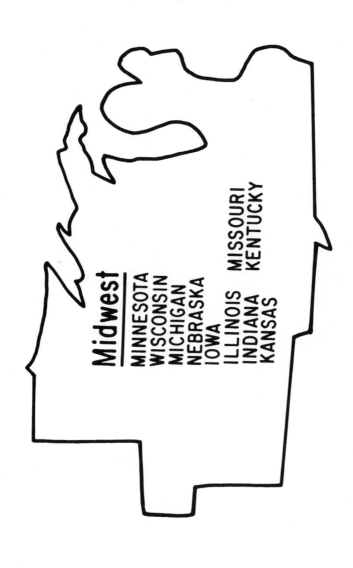

Midwest

MINNESOTA
WISCONSIN
MICHIGAN
NEBRASKA
IOWA
ILLINOIS
INDIANA
KANSAS
MISSOURI
KENTUCKY

Trees: Ash, Birch, Cottonwood, Elder, Elm, Oak
Grasses: Orchard grass, Redtop, Rye, Timothy
Weeds: Amaranthus spp., Lamb's Quarter, Plantain, Ragweed, Rumex spp., Russian thistle, Water hemp

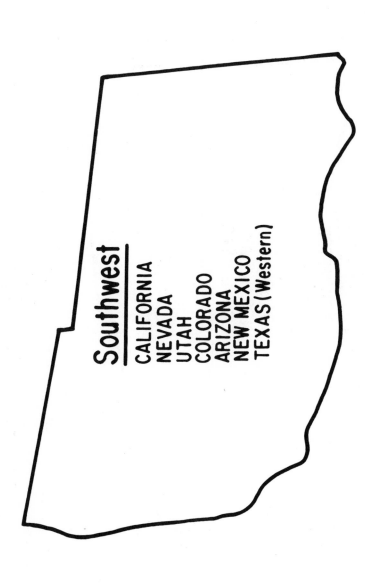

Southwest

CALIFORNIA
NEVADA
UTAH
COLORADO
ARIZONA
NEW MEXICO
TEXAS (Western)

Trees: Alder, Ash, Birch, Cedar, Cottonwood, Elder, Elm, Oak, Olive, Sycamore
Grasses: Bermuda grass, Brome, Fescue, Orchard grass, Poa spp., Redtop, Rye,
          Timothy   Sage, Saltbush
Weeds: Amaranthus spp., Cocklebur, Plantain, Ragweed, Rumex spp., Russian thistle,

30

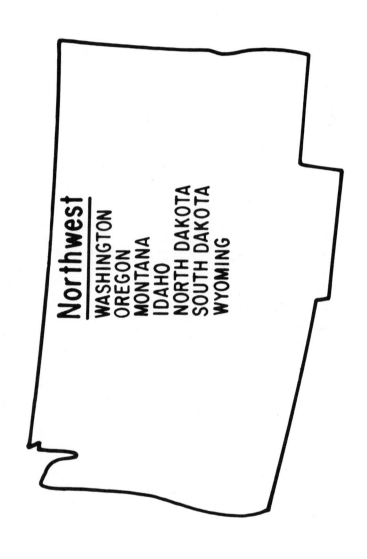

Northwest

WASHINGTON
OREGON
MONTANA
IDAHO
NORTH DAKOTA
SOUTH DAKOTA
WYOMING

Trees: Alder, Birch, Cottonwood, Elder, Elm, Oak
Grasses: Brome, Orchard grass, Poa spp., Redtop, Rye, Timothy
Weeds: Amaranthus spp., Lamb's Quarter, Plantain, Ragweed, Rumex spp., Sage brush, Saltbush

lation centers. Weather shows its effects on the cold-
er northern reaches of this region with conifers seen
commonly. This plant growth pattern is also seen on
the western slope of the Appalachian to its mergence
with the Ohio River Valley. Except for the Southern
end of the Appalachians, the Southeast U.S. is low and
level geographically with a temperate climate and moderate to heavy rainfall. Grasses are common. The
deciduous forests of the mountainous areas become mixed
as one approaches the coasts, an important consideration as conifer pollen is only locally important because of its weight.

The Midwestern states are well suited geographically
and climatically for the growth of grasses, native and
cultivated grains. Trees are less important in pollinosis except for isolated forests and cultivated stands.
Weeds may be very important particularly because of its
rapid invasion of fields left to fallow.

The Rocky Mountain States, with its high altitude,
low rainfall and cold climate, primarily supports conifers and low shrub growth, with a relative low pollen
distribution except in areas of population centers.

The arid Southwest with its warm summers has sparse
low shrub growth with trees and grasses surviving only
in areas where water is available such as river banks.

REFERENCES

Munz, P.A., Keck, D.D.: A California flora. Univ. of
   California Press. 1959.
Jepson, W.L.: A Manual of the flowering plants of Cal-
   ifornia. Sather Gate Bookshop, Berkeley, California
   1925.
Robins, W.W., Bellue, M.K., Ball, W.S.: Weeds of Cal-
   ifornia. Printing Division, California Dept. of
   Agriculture, 1951.
McMinn, H.E., Maino, E.: Pacific Coast Trees. Univ-
   ersity of California Press, 1937.
Ogden, EC, Raynor, GS, Hayes, JV, Lewis, DM & Haines,
   JH: Manual for sampling airborne pollen, New York,
   Hafner Press, 1974.

Stephen M. Nagy, Jr.

EVALUATION AND MANAGEMENT OF
CHRONIC NASAL SYMPTOMS

INTRODUCTION

Stuffy, runny noses rank amongst the most common complaints seen by primary physicians. Generally, there is a tendency to treat initial complaints with antihistamine decongestants, followed by an antibiotic when symptoms persist, especially with a purulent discharge. Then, if the patient returns again, frustration begins to set in. The following case summaries are of patients that presented to an allergist's office in May 1978 during what was an extremely severe pollen season.

All had been seen by their family physician who diagnosed inhalant, allergic disease. In fact, only one had significant pollen sensitivities.

1. A thirty-seven year old male complained of two months of significant nasal and sinus congestion, postnasal drip, rhinorrhea which was white and occasionally yellow. He had mild tenderness in his maxillary areas. There was minimal eye irritation and a nagging cough. His past medical history was totally unremarkable and past nasal and allergic history revealed only occasional upper respiratory infections, but no history of chronic or seasonal nasal symptoms. He had had eczema as an infant and had been taken off various foods.

2. A forty-seven year old female complains of severe nasal congestion for 2 months. There is a slight associated, non-productive cough, but there is no significant rhinorrhea and eye symptoms are quite minimal. She can recall some very minimal nasal symptoms in previous springs. Her past medical history includes diabetes (insulin dependence) for the last ten years and occasional elevations of blood pressure; anti-hypertensives were begun in January 1978. Her own past allergic

33

history is negative for any atopic problems in childhood.
   3. A twenty-two year old female has a two month
history of severe nasal congestion, a clear watery
rhinorrhea, sneezing, moderate itching of her nose and
eyes and a slight cough. The patient has experienced
similar symptoms for the last four to five springs.
They have usually cleared by June. This year the symptoms are much more severe. Her past medical history is
unremarkable. However, in childhood she had a history
of recurrent otitis and can recall that she was a chronic sniffler that seemed to clear by the time she complet-
ed grammar school.
   4. A twenty-eight year old male complains of
increased nasal congestion with minimal rhinorrhea but
with significant post-nasal drip for the last two to
three months. Close questioning reveals that the
patient has experienced mild nasal congestion which has
intermittently been worse for many years and which has
been associated with post-nasal drip. He is unsure,
but thinks that the symptoms might possibly have been
worse in the spring and the fall. He is also unsure as
to the total duration of his symptoms. The patient has
been quite healthy all of his life. Past allergic
history is negative for asthma or eczema, but as a child
he was taken off of milk for an unknown reason for two
years.
   Each of these cases will be discussed herein following formal consideration of the problem in general.
   Communication of disorders related to the nasal,
sinus and conjunctival areas frequently make use of
euphemisms such as "hay fever symptoms," "upper respiratory symptoms," and "sinus-type problem." This does
a disservice to the patient and the physician. First,
a patient should be encouraged to ennumerate his or her
specific complaints. Is the prime problem congestion
or significant rhinorrhea or both? Is the congestion
unilateral or bilateral, and is it confined solely to
the nose or is there a significant sense of pressure
within the maxillary and/or frontal sinus areas? What
is the nature of the discharge? If there is no significant anterior rhinorrhea, is there a significant post-
nasal drainage? Do the words congestion or fullness
adequately describe the patient's discomfort? Is the
prime symptom a pain or ache? Are there associated

conjunctival symptoms or palatal symptoms? Is the
nature of these symptoms primarily irritative or pruritic? Then, with a definition of terms, the physician
can adequately explore the chronology and temporal relationships. On close questioning, symptoms that were
initially presented as being acute may really have
existed for many years in a milder form. Associations
with specific environmental exposures such as animals,
house dust, windy days, mowing the lawn and specific
foods can then be explored with specific reference to
which symptoms are increased. Marked changes with
travel strongly suggest an inhalant etiology, as do
regular seasonal exacerbations.

      The family history should be explored for an atopic
background looking for a history in close family members
of infantile eczema, asthma, recurrent nasal symptoms,
and infant food sensitivities. The patient's past allergic history should also be explored for atopic problems, as well as for aspirin use and sensitivity. The
triad of asthma, nasal polyps and aspirin sensitivity
will be discussed in depth in another chapter. The past
medical history should pay particular attention to all
of the patient's current medications. Certain drugs
have as their commonest side effect, chronic nasal
symptoms and include reserpine, propanolol, and phenothiazines. The duration and frequency of nose drops or
sprays should be well documented. Such medication can
lead to a rhinitis medicamentosa and can be primarily
etiologic.

      The physical examination should note the color and
degree of swelling of the nasal membranes. Extreme
paleness and swelling is strongly indicative of an allergic inhalant etiology but is not pathognomonic.
Nasal polyps appear as greyish-white pearls and may be
so large as to actually totally protrude from the nostril. They may also be small and posterior and not be
visualized by an anterior exam. In extremely inhalant-
sensitive patients, the membrane may be so edematous as
to present a polypoid appearance. Swelling under the
eyes is a sign of chronic intranasal and/or sinus inflammation and if hyperpigmentation is present, it is
evidence of a problem of some months duration. Inflam-
ed conjunctival membranes should be noted. Marked
edema of the scleral conjunctivae is almost universally

seen in severe pollen allergy, especially in children.

TABLE 1
Classification of Etiology and Conditions Leading to
Chronic Nasal Symptoms
1. Inhalants: IgE or irritant mediated
2. Food "sensitivity": usually milk and probably not
    antibody mediated
3. Infectious
4. Iatrogenic, i.e. medications
5. Neoplasm: benign (polyps or granuloma) and malignant
6. Vasomotor syndrome
7. Anatomical poor airway in the absence of neoplasm
8. Histamine cephalgia
9. Cerebrospinal fluid rhinorrhea

INHALANTS

    These are the prime offenders in "allergic rhinitis"
and are usually classified as pollens, epidermals
(animals), molds and household (dust). Uncommonly,
foods such as grain, fish, or nuts are aerosolized and
produce symptoms by inhalation. The mechanism presumes
the presence of antigen-specific IgE antibody on tissue
mast cells within the nasal and conjunctival mucosa.
Contact with antigens leads to the release of histamine,
the major mediator, and is the reason why significant
itching of the nose, eyes, ears and palate is the hallmark of "allergic disease" and frequently helps differentiate it from other etiologies. Symptoms are almost
always worse on specific exposures such as mowing the
lawn, cleaning the attic, going into a musty cellar or
handling animals. They also remit when the antigen is
avoided as on trips or, in cases of occupational exposure, on weekends. Total IgE is usually significantly
elevated and skin tests should be positive to the specific offending antigens. Skin testing, however, is a
presumptive form of diagnosis as it "presumes" that the
IgE detected in the skin is present on the mast cells
of the nasal mucosa. For years allergists have identified and treated patients who have negative skin tests
but a positive correlative history. Only recent stud -
ies have indicated that there may be local production
of IgE within the nasal mucosa without it being detect-

able in the skin or serum.

Chemicals and even commonly used aerosols such as insecticides, deodorants or hair spray may cause significant symptoms simply as irritants. Of late, there has been considerable controversy as to a subset of patients who seem "sensitive" to the "chemical environment". We all know patients who are made quite ill by such exposures as exhaust fumes, excessively smoggy days and other chemicals previously noted. The mechanism, however, is obscure and is definitely not IgE mediated and their treatment with other than appropriate environmental control and symptomatic medications falls into the category of "unproven techniques".

FOODS

An acute anaphylactic reaction to a food may well have nasal congestion, clear rhinorrhea, and itching as part of the spectrum of symptoms. In these cases, skin tests might well detect IgE antibody to the offending food. However, the mechanism by which various foods, particularly milk, produce chronic nasal congestion and rhinorrhea is unclear. Nevertheless, we are all familiar with children with severe nasal congestion, chronic sniffling, rubbing of the nose and large "allergic shiners"; such patients often respond dramatically to the elimination of milk or other food, i.e. wheat, corn, chocolate, tomatoes, eggs. These symptoms are not uncommon in adults; however, the congestion is usually not as prominent and the "shiners" are absent. Such patients present with chronic mild to moderate nasal congestion and usually post-nasal discharge, which, on close questioning, has usually been present for many years in varying severity. Not unusually, their past allergic history reveals colic or some other form of milk intolerance in infancy. Skin testing is almost universally useless in diagnosis which can best be done by an appropriate elimination diet. Finally, treatment consists of simple dietary restriction.

INFECTIOUS

Upper respiratory infections are almost always caused by viruses and are self-limited and should not

lead to chronic nasal symptoms. In fact, the recurrent
diagnosis of acute viral respiratory infections should
lead one to search for a non-infectious cause. Nonetheless, chronic sinusitis, unlike acute sinusitis, may
present as simply chronic nasal obstruction with a chronic clear discharge. The other signs of acute sinusitis
such as fever, purulent discharge and significant unilateral or bilateral maxillary tenderness with perior-
bital edema may be absent. The usual history is that of
a URI several weeks to several months previously that
simply did not resolve. In fact, the number of patients
that present with a several year history of "recurrent
allergies" and who, in fact, have bilateral maxillary
fluid levels is significant. A variant of this syndrome
is a total absence of nasal or sinus symptoms and simply
a severe chronic cough, or even asthma. The diagnosis
is made by appropriate paranasal sinus films. The physician should not depend on transillumination. Treatment consists of decongestants and antibiotics. If
unsuccessful, antral irrigation and appropriate drainage procedures may be indicated, particularly in long-
standing cases. An infectious etiology, however, does
not preclude an allergic diathesis which may be an important predisposing factor.

RHINITIS MEDICAMENTOSA

     This appellation is frequently reserved for the
chronic nasal obstruction that is experienced by
patients who abuse or are addicted to local nasal decongestants. These sympathomimetics are locally extremely
irritating and histologically lead to disruption of the
basement membrane. Although they are usually begun for
an acute process, when used over one to two weeks, they
themselves can become primarily etiologic with the
patient caught in the cycle. Attempts to get the
patient off the drops by strong verbal persuasion will
probably lead to poor compliance; what is really required is a medication that will, in fact, lead to a clear-
er nasal passage. This usually takes the form of a
steroid aerosol and, if that fails, a short course of
oral steroids to be gradually tapered. Such patients
require frequent follow-up to ensure the drops are discontinued.

Probably the commonest oral medication to cause
significant nasal symptomatology is the Rauwolfia alk-
loid, reserpine. It is used almost exclusively in hypertension. Pharmacologically it depletes stores of cate-
cholamines and 5HT in many organs and the pharmacological effects are attributed to this action. Characteristically, the blood pressure drops gradually over several
weeks, presumably because the depletion is also a gradual process. For this reason, the nasal congestion,
which is the commonest side effect of reserpine, is frequently insidious and not even noted until several weeks
or even months after the initiation of reserpine therapy.
Also, there are so many combination antihypertensives,
the consulting physician may not even realize the
patient is on reserpine unless the drug is produced.
Just as the onset is gradual, so do the symptoms slowly
improve with discontinuation of therapy; one should wait
at least six weeks before looking for other etiologies.
The beta blocker, propanolol, used frequently in ar-
rythmias and with increasing frequency in hypertension,
produces fairly dramatic nasal congestion. It is more
notoriously known, however, for its exacerbation of
bronchial asthma. Improvement with discontinuation is
usually more rapid. The phenothiazines, particularly
thoridazine (Mellaril), produce a nasal dryness and congestion without significant rhinorrhea that is quite
uncomfortable. Unfortunately, there are no good alternatives and treatment of the underlying psychotic or
neurotic disorder may take precedence. Chronic aspirin
useage may produce syndromes of chronic profuse rhinorrhea and minimal nasal congestion. More specifically,
patients with polyps may have an increased sensitivity
to aspirin which is non-immunologic; part of that sensitivity may be manifested by increased nasal symptoms.

NEOPLASM

Malignant lesions of the nasopharynx, nasal antra,
and sinuses may present with increasing obstruction and
particularly with chronic recurrent epistaxis. Nasal
polyps are the commonest benign neoplasm and are easily
diagnosed as pearly gray excrescences within the nasal
antra. However, they may be present only posteriorly
and not be visible by anterior exam. In extremely

severe pollenosis, the nasal mucosa may be so edematous
as to give the appearance of polyps. Histologically,
the polyps are full of eosinophiles; a nasal smear will
show extensive numbers of these cells even in non-atopic
disease.

VASOMOTOR SYNDROME

This category defines a subset of patients that seem
excessively responsive to certain stimuli such as
changes in temperature, chemical irritants, and occasionally stress and alcohol. Such patients are usually
"non-allergic"; however, there may be a vasomotor component to an allergic rhinitis. The presumed abnormality is increased sensitivity of neural receptors within
the nose. Such patients have perennial symptoms of both
nasal obstruction and/or rhinorrhea. The importance of
the diagnosis is to avoid immunotherapy. Such patients
also frequently undergo surgical procedures with poor
results.

ANATOMICAL POOR AIRWAY

In all of the above, the nasal obstruction is presumed due to mucosal swelling. Such patients give histories of complete clearing of symptoms, either spontaneously, with season, or with treatment, especially with
short courses of corticosteroids. There is a group of
patients who present with primarily nasal obstruction,
usually with minimal nasal discharge, in whom the obstruction is almost constant. Marked septal deformity
due to either previous trauma or even long-standing
severe allergic rhinitis may progress to the point where
the obstruction will be relieved only by surgical intervention. Such a diagnosis is appropriately made by a
qualified otolaryngologist.

HISTAMINE CEPHALGIA (Horton's Headache)

This syndrome of questionable etiology is characterized by unilateral nasal congestion followed by profuse
rhinorrhea and unilateral lacrimation associated with
throbbing headaches on the ipsalateral side. Occasionally, there is ptosis, meiosis, and edema of the cheek,

although there are usually no other signs of histamine
release such as marked sneezing or itching. It is
classically nocturnal, tending to occur nightly for
weeks or months, with long intervals of freedom (hence
the name "cluster" headaches).

CEREBROSPINAL FLUID RHINORRHEA

     This is a rare entity, but one which must be borne
in mind in the patient with chronic or intermittent unilateral clear nasal discharge. It results from a fistu-
lous connection, usually traumatic, between the frontal
or ethmoid sinuses and the subarachnoid space. It also
predisposes to recurrent attacks of bacterial meningitis.
The diagnosis is usually made by introducing a tracer,
either a dye or radioactive material, into the cerebrospinal fluid and detecting it in nasal secretions. A
glucose determination of the discharge may be helpful
since generally glucose is minimal or absent in the
normal mucus secretions, but approximates cerebrospinal
fluid glucose in this disorder.

DIAGNOSTIC PROCEDURES

SKIN TESTING

     Skin tests have been the hallmark of "allergic"
evaluations since their introduction sixty to seventy
years ago. They represent an exposure to various suspected antigens and confirm the presence of antigen
specific IgE. Patients should not take classical antihistamines for forty-eight to seventy-two hours nor
hydroxyzine (Atarax, Vistaril) and hydroxyzine containing preparations (Marax) for at least four days prior to
testing. Additionally, the antigens selected for testing should be based in part on the history and the local
flora. Food testing, although possibly helpful in acute
reactions, is virtually worthless when dealing with
chronic nasal symptoms. Anaphylactic reactions are rare
but definitely possible and a physician should be readily available.
     The three primary types of testing are scratch,
prick and intradermal methods. Scratch testing utilizes
scarafiers to abrade the skin; a drop of concentrated

TABLE 2
Historical and laboratory characterization of chronic nasal symptoms

	Characteristic Symptoms	Skin Tests	Nasal Smear for Eosinophiles	IgE	Sinus Films
Inhalants	Seasonal, severe itching	Usually positive	Very positive	Usu. Elev.	Neg.
Foods		Not helpful	Negative	Normal	Neg.
Infectious	Usually purulent discharge, occasional fever	Negative	Occasionally positive	Normal	Pos.
Iatrogenic		Negative	Negative	Normal	Neg.
Neoplasm	Epistaxis is common if malignant	Polyps may be assoc. w̄ atopy & pos. tests.	Very positive w̄ nasal polyps	Elev. if polyps assoc. w̄ atopy	Usu. Pos.
Vasomotor Syndrome		Negative	Negative	Normal	Neg.
Poor Airway	Primarily severe nasal congestion	May be pos.	Occasionally positive	Occas. Elev.	Neg.

| Histamine Cephalgia | Usually clear discharge | Negative | Negative | Normal | Neg. |
| Cerebrospinal Fluid Rhinorrhea | Usually clear discharge | Negative | Negative | Normal | Neg. |

water-extracted antigen and glycerine is then applied.
Because of the high concentration anaphylactic reactions
are probably commonest with this technique. It is suggested that as soon as a positive reaction occurs
the remaining antigen be removed from the skin, i.e.
erased, to reduce this probability. While scratch testing normally is performed on the skin of the back,
intradermal tests are usually placed on the volar surface of the lower or upper arm. Approximately 0.02 ml
of fluid is injected with a 26 gauge needle into the
dermis so that a small bleb is formed. The concentration of the antigen will vary depending upon the technique employed. Many allergists screen their patients
with scratch testing, then utilize intradermal testing
if the latter are negative or equivocal. End point
titration testing with this technique is probably the
most sensitive when compared to case histories. Prick
testing consists of applying a drop of solution to the
skin test site, usually the back, and passing a 26 gauge
needle through the drop into the skin. The concentration utilized is greater than in intradermal testing
and less than in scratch testing. The methods of grading these reactions vary. Usually a system involving
an arbitrary division of 1+ to 4+ based on the amount
of erythema and the size of the wheal is employed for
scratch and intradermal testing. In prick testing, the
wheal and erythema are simply measured without any grading taking place. An appropriate diluent control and a
histamine control should be performed with each set of
testing. This rules out significant dermatographism in
the former and probable antihistamine use in the latter.
     Although these studies are invaluable when perform-
ed properly, it cannot be over-emphasized that it takes
a great deal of skill and experience to be consistent in
results and interpretation. At times erythema maybe
due to irritative properties, improper technique or
simply hypersensitive skin. The importance of stating
that a test is positive is critical since it labels the
patient "allergic" and determines which antigens are to
be avoided and, in some instances, the ones to which he
will be immunized. It is therefore not a procedure to
be entered into on an infrequent basis by untrained
personnel.

RAST

The RAST (Radio-Allergosorbent Test) measures antigen specific IgE in the serum by a radio-immunoassay.
It has become increasingly popular over the last several years and, in large part, this is due to the drawbacks of skin testing outlined above. The specific
measurement, unlike skin testing, does not vary with
technique. This brief discussion will not enter into
the controversy of its reliability as compared to skin
testing. Suffice it to say that it is probably as sensitive as competently performed skin tests. It is
specifically indicated in situations where:
1. patients have experienced anaphylactic reactions to
    skin testing,
2. where the skin is so involved in a dermatopathic
    process that skin testing is not feasible, or
3. in the extremely young infant whom the physician
    does not want to traumatize.
RAST drawbacks have included cost, a several week
delay in obtaining results, and a limited battery of
antigens.

SINUS FILMS

This is one of the few diagnostic procedures that is
under-utilized. Transillumination is not an adequate
means of determining the presence or absence of fluid
and gives no idea as to longstanding chronic changes
without fluid. In the chronically afflicted patient,
in whom the etiology is not obviously apparent, i.e.
reserpine, flagrant pollinosis, they should be almost
routine. The high level of pathology associated with
the older asthmatic, nasal polyps and aspirin sensitivity virtually require them. Unfortunately, there is
an unevenness of both quality of roentgengrams and interpretation even among qualified radiologists. One
must be wary of such reports as "faint haziness" of
maxillary antra and should demand more definable criteria such as the presence or absence of fluid and/or
the presence or absence and degree of mucosal thickening.

TOTAL IgE

This represents an excellent screening tool to detect atopic patients. It is important to emphasize,
however, that if one is going to skin test the patient
or obtain a number of RAST procedures, then a concomitant total IgE is probably superfluous. In children,
however, a negative battery of scratch tests to inhalants in the presence of a significantly elevated total
IgE might lead one to perform selective intradermals.
Elevations of total IgE have been correlated with extrinsic asthma and hay fever. The level is higher if
there are multiple allergies as opposed to a single
allergy. This will have significant clinical correlations since severe perennial symptomatology might result
from solitary sensitivities to specific animals or
molds, yet the total IgE may be normal or only slightly
elevated. Mold allergy in general also produces very
low levels of IgE. Markedly elevated levels are
found in helminthic infections, IgE myeloma, and in
eczema with other associated diseases. In "pure"
eczema without respiratory symptoms, IgE concentrations
are usually normal.

NASAL SMEARS

Although eosinophilia either in serum or in secretions has been a hallmark of allergic disease, its
marked predominance in the sputa of severe intrinsic
asthmatics, in non-allergic nasal polyps and its intermittent appearance in infectious rhinosinusitis proves
that one cannot use it to distinguish atopic from non-
atopic disease. The nasal smear is usually obtained
by having the patient blow his nose into heavy waxed
paper. The secretions can then be examined and subsequently transferred to a slide and stained with either
Wright's or Hansel's stain. Grading by laboratories is
usually based on one plus to four plus depending on the
percentage and number of eosinophiles present. In the
absence of nasal polyps and frank sinusitis, a positive
smear would certainly make an allergic etiology quite
likely. However, the absence of eosinophiles does not
rule out that diagnosis. It is probably most helpful
as a screening procedure in patients with perennial

non-seasonal symptoms and the absence of other obvious
etiologies.

CASE DISCUSSIONS

1. This thirty-seven year old male had bilateral maxillary fluid levels and responded quite well to antibiotics and decongestants. His skin tests were completely negative and the onset of his illness in the
spring was quite fortuitous.
2. This forty-seven year old female had been started
on reserpine for her hypertension. It reveals that
patients with chronic nasal symptoms can be very sug-
gestable when in the midst of other classically "allergic" patients.
3. This twenty-two year old female is the only classical atope. She experienced a typical pattern of chronic
allergic rhinitis in childhood, clearing by adolescence,
and for an unknown reason, made its appearance again in
the late teens and early twenties.
4. This twenty-eight year old male had a dramatic response to a milk-free diet. He, too, like so many
patients with chronic nasal symptoms, was very suggest-
ible primarily because, in the eyes of the layman, the
major etiology of chronic symptoms is inhalants.

TREATMENT

     Allergic management can be somewhat complicated
utilizing various medications, environmental measures,
and possibly immunotherapy. For this reason, two separate chapters of this volume have been devoted to this.
The treatment of the other entities is more straightforward providing it is a solitary problem and the diagnosis is certain. Unfortunately, in many patients,
a single diagnosis is not appropriate. Inhalant
allergy may be combined with food sensitivity; infectious and allergic problems are complicated by the
concomitant use of medications. Frequently, a diagnosis is made only as a result of various therapeutic
regimens.

REFERENCES

Taylor, M: The origin and functions of nasal mucus,
    Laryngoscope 84:612, 1974.
Proctor, DF, Andersen, I, Lundqvist, G: Clearance of
    inhaled particles from the human nose, Arch. Intern.
    Med. 131:132, 1973.
Drettner, B.:   Pathophysiological relationship between
    the upper and lower airways, Ann. Otol. Rhinol.
    Laryngol. 79: 499, 1970.
Norman, PS: The clinical significance of IgE, Hosp.
    Prac. 10:41, 1975.
Samter M, Durham, OC: Regional allergy of the United
    States, Canada, Mexico and Cuba. Springfield, Ill.
    Charles C Thomas, 1955.
Levy DA, Lichtenstein, LM, Goldstein, EO, Ishizaka, K:
    Immunologic and cellular changes accompanying the
    therapy of pollen allergy. J Clin Invest 50:360,
    1971.

Michael H. Keslin

ANTIHISTAMINE, SYMPATHOMIMETIC
AGENTS AND STEROID TREATMENT OF
ALLERGIC RHINITIS

INTRODUCTION

Allergic rhinitis accounted for 11,417,000 private
patient visits during the year 1975 according to stat-
istics collected by the National Disease and Therapeutic Index Report. Because almost all primary care
physicians are involved in the treatment of these patients it is important for primary care physicians as
well as allergists and other specialists to be familiar
with the therapy of this disease.

GENERAL THERAPEUTIC CONSIDERATIONS

There are several levels of therapy in the management of allergic rhinitis (Table 1). The first level
of therapy includes environmental control measures to
reduce dust, feathers, mold, pet dander and pollen.
Dust avoidance precautions include frequent vacuuming
of the patient's bedroom and removal of clutter and
nicknacks which might collect dust. If feather pillows are used it is worthwhile to obtain rubberized plastic zipper covers. Similarly mattress covers should
be used if the mattress or box spring are old. Fortunately these are usually unnecessary with most modern
mattresses and box springs. Mold avoidance precautions
include elimination of obvious sources of mold, such
as old or peeling wallpaper or linoleum. In addition
it is helpful to spray bathrooms, under sinks, service
areas and window sills with fungicidal agents such as
Zephiran chloride*. Patients should also avoid areas

*17% concentrate diluted with an equal volume of water
and used in a hand sprayer twice a week.

of heavy mold concentration such as barns, old leaves
or basements. If patients are sensitive to pets, the
animals should be kept out of doors or restricted to a
small area of the house. The animals should never be
in the patient's bedroom. It is helpful to keep the
bedroom windows closed at night, particularly during
the pollen season. Heavy pollen exposure can occur
during sleep if this is not done. Furthermore it is
important for patients with allergic rhinitis not to
smoke. Air filters or purifiers are sometimes helpful
in decreasing the concentration of pollens or dust in
the house. The second level of allergic rhinitis
therapy includes the use of various medications. The
most useful drugs are antihistamines, sympathomimetic
agents, or intranasal corticosteroid sprays. The
third level of allergic rhinitis treatment includes
the use of specific immunotherapy. This is discussed
in detail on page 109.

ANTIHISTAMINES

Antihistamines represent a diverse group of compounds which antagonize various actions of the chemical histamine. Histamine is synthesized in the body
from L-histadine by the enzyme -histadine decarboxy-
lase. Histamine is stored in mast cells and basophils
as a complex with heparin in membrane limited secretory granules. When mast cells are depleted of histamine stores, it may take weeks for these stores to be
repleted. Some free histamine is present in the epi-
dermis, central nervous system, and gastrointestinal
mucoke. Brisk turnover and release of histamine occurs
in these latter sites. The major pharmacological effects of histamine include the following:

a) Cardiovascular system - capillary dilatation is
the most important action of histamine on the cardiovascular system in man. This results from direct action of histamine on the walls of vessels in
the microcirculation. Increased capillary permeability results from direct effect of histamine on
postcapillary venules. The endothelial cells of
these vessels separate at their boundaries and in-

crease permeability to plasma proteins and fluid.
The plasma proteins and fluid are then free to
pass into the extracellular space, resulting in
edema formation.

b) Respiratory system - histamine can cause intense
bronchoconstriction in asthmatics by direct action
on bronchial smooth muscle cells. Histamine seems
to cause little bronchoconstriction in nonasthmatic
subjects.

c) Exocrine glands - histamine stimulates parietal
and chief cells to secrete acid and pepsin. Some
stimulation of salivary, pancreatic, intestinal,
bronchial and lacrimal glands also occurs but this
seems to be of little importance in man.

d) Sensory nerve endings - the "flare" component of
the triple response is a result of the direct stimulation of nerve endings by histamine. When histamine is injected into the skin, a small, red spot
a few mm. in diameter develops within seconds and
reaches maximum size in one minute. Then a red
flush or "flare" slowly develops and may extend 10
mm. from the latter original red spot. This represents the "flare" component of the triple response. Localized edema fluid develops about 90
seconds after injection and comes to occupy the
site of the original red spot. The first component of the response is due to local dilatation of
minute blood vessels, but the flare is due to widespread dilatation of neighboring arterioles mediated through local axon reflex mechanisms. The
third component or wheal formation is due to increased permeability of fine blood vessels. Finally, histamine may cause pain and itching following deep intradermal administration.

These varied effects of histamine are mediated by
direct stimulation of specific receptor sites. It is
now known that there are at least two specific types
of receptor sites for histamine. H_1 receptor sites are
operationally defined as those receptors responsible

for all effects of histamine blocked by the so-called
classical (pre-1972) antihistamine drugs. These drugs,
however, do not interfere with histamine stimulant
effects on gastric secretion, the heart, or the rela-
xant effect on isolated rat uterus and sheep bronchus.
Certain effects of histamine such as vasodilatation and
edema formation seem to involve synergistic stimulation
of both H_1 and H_2 receptor sites. H_2 receptor blockers
such as cimetidine, are effective in blocking gastric
secretion.

    Antihistamines are a diverse group of compounds
containing an ethylamine ($CH_2-CH_2-N=$) side chain which
resembles that of histamine. The side chain is attach-
ed to a cyclic or heterocyclic ring which may be a py-
ridine, piperadine, pyrrolidine, piperazine, phenothiazine or even an imidazole group. These drugs can be
partially classified on the basis of the linkage between the ethylamine group and the large basic radicals.
The linkage to the ethylamine structure may contain a
nitrogen, oxygen or carbon atom. If the linkage group
is nitrogen, then the compounds are classified as
ethylenediamine derivatives; if the linkage group is
oxygen, then the compounds are classified as ethanola-
mines; and if the linkage group is a carbon atom, then
the compounds are classified as alkylamines. Compounds
with cyclic structures are classified as piperazines
and phenothiazines.
    Table 2 outlines representative examples of anti-
histamine derivatives from each of the five basic
classes of antihistamines (H_1 blockers) and also shows
the relationship of these drugs to histamine. Cimetadine and metiamide, two of the new H_2 receptor blocker drugs are also pictured. Metiamide however is no
longer widely used because of reports of agranulocytosis
in a few patients. This has not been a problem with
cimetadine which is now used for treatment of Zollinger-
Ellison syndrome and peptic ulcer disease.
    All five classes of H_1 receptor blockers have simi-
lar efficacy as histamine antagonists, but vary somewhat in potency, dosage and relative incidence of side
effects. In general antihistamines, in the ethanolamine group, have a marked tendency to cause sedation
and atropine-like activity. They have little in the

way of GI side effects. Ethylenediamines cause little
central nervous system depression but frequently cause
GI side effects. Alkylamines seem to be quite effective in relatively low doses and have been found to be
most useful in the treatment of allergic rhinitis because of the low incidence of side effects. Piperazines and phenothiazines frequently cause sedation and
only a few drugs in these categories have been found
useful in the treatment of allergic rhinitis. There
is significant individual variation in the efficacy of
a given antihistamine and its accompanying side effects.
It is best to try a few representative drugs from each
class in a given patient and choose the drug which
causes the best clinical response with the least undesirable side effects. Occasionally, patients will
become tolerant to a given antihistamine and it may
be useful to try another drug, either in the same class
or from another class. Usually it is better to use a
single drug in adequate doses than to use several
drugs in smaller doses.

     About 25% of patients will develop significant
side effects from various antihistamine preparations.
These side effects can be classified as follows:
     a) Central action: Sedation, dizziness, tinnitus,
     lassitude, incoordination, fatigue, blurred vision,
     diplopia, euphoria, nervousness, insomnia and
     tremors.
     b) Gastrointestinal System: Anorexia, nausea, vo-
     miting, epigastric distress, constipation, and
     diarrhea. It seems best to give the drugs with
     meals in an effort to try to minimize these GI
     side effects.
     c) Cardiorespiratory System: Dryness of the mouth,
     throat, and respiratory passages can develop. Pal-
     pitations, hypotension and tightness of the chest
     have also been reported.
     d) Genitourinary System: Urinary frequency
     e) Allergic Reactions: Rarely occur from systemic
     administration of antihistamines. More common is
     allergic contact dermatitis secondary to topical
     application of antihistamines. Consequently this
     route of administration has essentially been aban-
     doned.

Table 3 outlines the duration of action, available
preparations, and usual adult dosage for representative
antihistamines in each of the five major classes. The
usual duration of action of these drugs is between four
and six hours. Chlorpheniramine maleate and bromphen-
iramine maleate are two of the most useful drugs for
the treatment of allergic rhinitis. Often doses in the
range of 4 mgs. two to four times a day will prove
quite effective in controlling some of the major symptoms of allergic rhinitis such as sneezing, rhinorrhea
and nasal pruritus. Antihistamines are less effective
in controlling nasal obstruction and allergic conjunc-
tivitis type symptoms. These drugs seem most effective when they are administered on a regular basis
throughout the pollen season rather than on an as
needed basis for symptomatic treatment. This observation is a reflection of the fact that antihistamines
function as competitive inhibitors of histamine, but
do not interfere with the release of histamine.

Acute antihistamine poisoning is typified by hal-
lucinations, excitement, ataxia, incoordination, atheto-
sis and convulsions. Fixed, dilated pupils, flushed
face and fever are common. Twenty-thirty tablets or
capsules of most commercially available antihistamine
represent a lethal or near-lethal dose for a small
child. There is no specific therapy for antihistamine
poisoning. Convulsions are treated with short acting
depressants, such as thiopental or diazepam.

Greenberger *et al* have recently reviewed the use of
various anti-allergy medications during pregnancy.
Their data indicates that there is no overall evidence
incriminating antihistamines as teratogenic during
pregnancy. They further state that judicious use of
diphenhydramine, tripelennamine, pheniramine, and
chlorpheniramine is safe during pregnancy. Piperazine
drugs such as chlorcyclizine however should be avoided
since teratogenic effects have been reported in laboratory animals. In general it seems best to use as
small a dose of medication as possible and to avoid
using any drugs during the early stages of pregnancy.

SYMPATHOMIMETIC AGENTS

Sympathomimetic drugs mimic the alpha-adrenergic

stimulant effect of epinephrine or norepinephrine.
These drugs are frequently combined with antihistamines
in various fixed dose combination pills in an effort to
better treat the nasal congestion associated with allergic rhinitis and also to counteract some of the so-
porific effect of the antihistamine drugs. Representative antihistamine/sympathomimetic combinations are
outlined in Table 4. Many of these drugs seem to be
quite helpful in symptomatic control of allergic rhinitis. Co-Pyronil is particularly helpful in some
patients with headaches secondary to allergic sinus
congestion. Ornade and Dimetapp work well for control
of most of the symptoms of allergic rhinitis. Actifed
is also quite useful although it seems to be somewhat
more likely to cause drowsiness. Disophrol or Drixoral
seem to be helpful in patients with severe nasal congestion.

Sympathomimetic nose drops or nose sprays should only
be used for the treatment of allergic rhinitis on a
very temporary basis. Prolonged use of these preparations may result in rhinitis medicamentosa which is
characterized by rebound vasodilatation after initial
vasoconstriction. This results in a vicious cycle of
more frequent use of the nose drop or nose spray followed by rapid onset of renewed nasal congestion. Often a
short course of Turbinaire Decadron is helpful in wean-
ing patients off nose sprays.

INTRANASAL STEROIDS

Dexamethasone sodium phosphate (Turbinaire) spray
has been found to decrease allergic rhinitis type symptoms in about 75% of patients with hay fever symptoms.
The usual dose is two whiffs in each nostril three
times a day which delivers approximately 0.96 mgs. of
dexamethasone. Turbinaire has also been demonstrated
to be effective in shrinking nasal polyps and as noted
previously, can be helpful in treating "rebound" phenomenon from overuse of sympathomimetic nasal sprays.
It is contraindicated in the presence of systemic fungal infections, hypersensitivity to dexamethasone or
any of the components of the spray, tuberculosis, viral and fungal nasal conditions and ocular herpes sim-
plex.

The main factor limiting the prolonged use of dexamethasone spray is the potential development of adrenal suppression. Norman *et al* studied seven patients
with ragweed hay fever treated with two sprays of Turbinaire three times a day during the ragweed pollen
season. They collected 24 hour urine specimens to
determine the excretion of 17-hydroxycorticosteroids.
Adrenal suppression was demonstrated in five of these
seven patients using this parameter. Two to three
weeks after discontinuation of the Turbinaire, excretion of 17-hydroxycorticosteroids was normal or near
normal in all but one patient. Because of the possibility of adrenal suppression, it is best to limit
courses of treatment with Turbinaire to a total of 10-
14 days. This often is enough to help control allergic
rhinitis symptoms during the height of the pollen season. A repeat course of treatment might be safely
undertaken within 3-4 weeks. A patient who has been on
Turbinaire, however, and undergoes the stress of surgery or trauma, might require replacement of gluco-
and mineralocorticoids.

Beclomethasone dipropionate is an inhaled corticosteroid available for the treatment of asthma in
the United States. This drug, marketed under the trade
name of Beconase in the United Kingdom, has been found
to be quite useful in treatment of allergic rhinitis.
Blair has recently reported a series of 20 patients
who demonstrated both subjective and objective improvement in perennial allergic rhinitis with Beconase therapy. Doses up to 400 micrograms per day have been demonstrated not to cause adrenal suppression. The usual
recommended dose for allergic rhinitis therapy is one
spray in each nostril twice a day (200 micrograms per
day). Beclomethasone nasal spray is not yet available
for use in the United States.

CONCLUSION

It must be emphasized that treatment for patients
should be an individualized decision. Moreover conservative management, i.e. environment control, is a
critical and often overlooked avenue. Indeed the most
judicious programs are a balance of therapeutic decisions, all geared on the basis of clinical severity

and response.

TABLE 1
Therapy of Allergic Rhinitis
I.   Environmental Control Measures
       A. Dust, Mold, Animals
       B. Windows Closed During Pollen Season
       C. Stop Smoking
       D. Air Filters or Purifiers

II.   Medical Therapy
       A. Antihistamines
       B. Decongestants
       C. Dexamethasone Nasal Spray (Turbinaire)

III.   Immunotherapy (Allergy Injections)

REFERENCES

Sheldon, JM, et al: A survey and evaluation of the
    antihistamine drugs, Bull. Am. Soc. Hosp. Pharma-
    cist 7:252, 1950.
Austen, KF, Lichtenstein, LM: Asthma, physiology, im-
    munopharmacology, and treatment. Aca. Press, New
    York, 1973.
Ahlquist, RP: A study of adrenotropic receptors, Am.
    J. Physiol. 153:586-600, 1948.
Lands, AM, et al: Differentiation of receptor systems
    activated by sympathmimetic amines, Nature 214:597-
    598, 1967.
Jenne, JW, et al: Pharmacokinetics of theophylline,
    Clin. Pharmacol. and Thera., 13:349-360, 1972.
Epstein, SE, Braunwald, E: Beta-adrenergic receptor
    blocking drugs, N.E.J.M., 275:1104-1112, 1966.
Piafsky, KM, Ogilvie, RI: Drug therapy: Dosage of
    theophylline in bronchial asthma, N.E.J.M., 292:
    1218-1222, 1975.
Chen, JO, et al: Sod. Cromoglycate, a new compound for
    the prevention of exacerbation of asthma, J.
    Allergy 43:89-100, 1969.
Webb-Johnson, Andrews, JL: Drug therapy: Bronchodila-
    tor therapy, N.E.J.M., 297:476-482, 758-764, 1977.

TABLE 2: REPRESENTATIVE ANTIHISTAMINES

Histamine:
$$HC\!\!=\!\!C-CH_2-CH_2-NH_2$$

(imidazole ring: HN, N, CH)

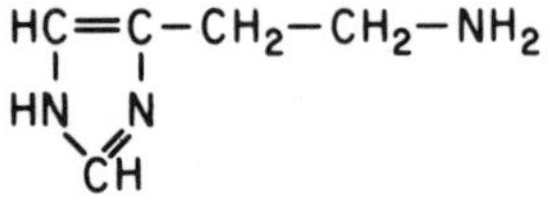

H_1-RECEPTOR ANTAGONISTS

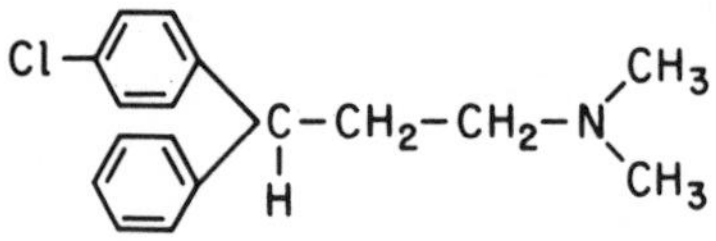

Alkylamine: chlorpheniramine

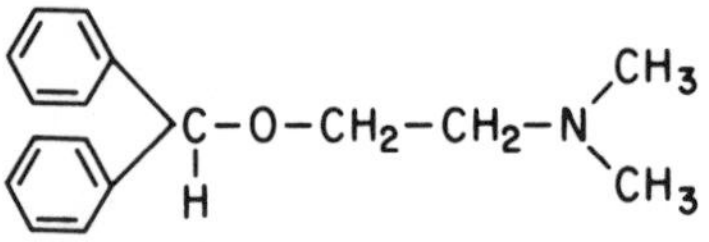

Cl—(phenyl)—$C-CH_2-CH_2-N(CH_3)(CH_3)$, with H and phenyl

Ethanolamine: diphenhydramine

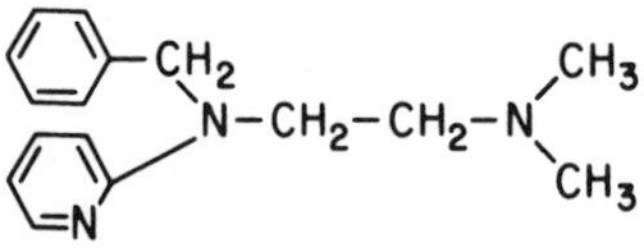

(diphenyl)$C-O-CH_2-CH_2-N(CH_3)(CH_3)$, with H

Ethylenediamine: tripelennamine

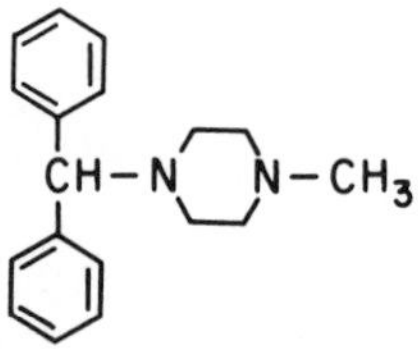

(phenyl)CH_2, (pyridine-N)$N-CH_2-CH_2-N(CH_3)(CH_3)$

Piperazine: cyclizine

(diphenyl)$CH-N$(piperazine)$N-CH_3$

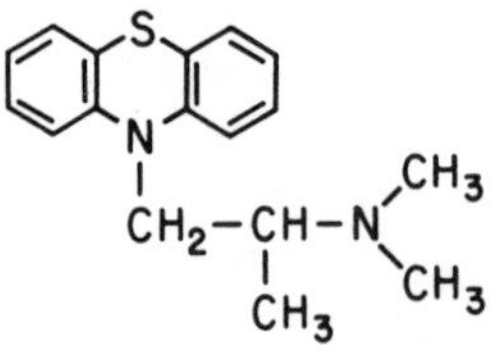

Phenothiazine: promethazine

(phenothiazine, S, N)$CH_2-CH-N(CH_3)(CH_3)$, with CH_3

H_2-RECEPTOR ANTAGONISTS

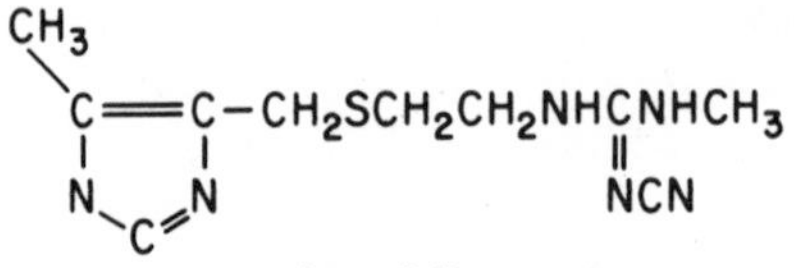

Cimetidine

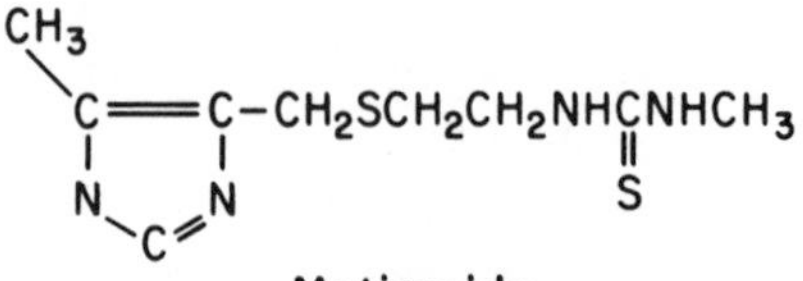

CH_3
$C\!\!=\!\!C-CH_2SCH_2CH_2NHCNHCH_3$
(imidazole: N, C, N) with $\underset{\parallel}{NCN}$

Metiamide

CH_3
$C\!\!=\!\!C-CH_2SCH_2CH_2NHCNHCH_3$
(imidazole: N, C, N) with $\underset{\parallel}{S}$

TABLE 3
Representative H_1 Blocking Antihistamines

Class and Non-Proprietary Name	Trade Name	Duration of Action (Hours)
Ethanolamines		
Diphenhydramine Hydrochloride	Benadryl	4-6
Dimehydrinate	Dramamine	4-6
Carbinoxamine Maleate	Clistin	3-4
Ethylenediamines		
Tripelennamine Hydrochloride	Pyribenzamine	4-6
Tripelennamine	Pyribenzamine	
Pyrilamine Maleate	Histalon, Neo-Antergan, Neo-Pyramine, Nisaval	4-6
Antazoline	Vasocor-A	3-4
Methapyrilene Hydrochloride	Histadyl	4-6
Alkylamines		
Chlorpheniramine Maleate	Chlor-Trimeton & many others	4-6
Brompheniramine Maleate	Dimetane	4-6
Piperazines		
Cyclizine Hydrochloride	Marezine	4-6
Cyclizine Lactate	Marezine	4-6
Meclizine Hydrochloride	Bonine	12-24
Phenothiazines		
Promethazine Hydrochloride	Phenergan	4-6

60

TABLE 4

Representative Antihistamine - Sympathomimetic
  Combinations

Trade Name	Ingredients	*Mg. Per Capsule or Tablet
Actifed	Triprolidine	2.5
	d-Isoephedrine	60
Co-pyronil	Pyrrobutamine	15
	Methapyrilene	25
	Cyclopentamine	12.5
Dallergy	Chlorpheniramine	8
	Phenylephrine	20
	Methscopolamine	2.5
Deconamine	Chlorpheniramine	8
	d-Pseudoephrine	120
Dimetapp	Brompheniramine	12
	Phenylpropanolamine	15
	Phenylephrine	15
Disophrol	Dexbrompheniramine	6
Drixoral	d-Isoephedrine	120
Extendryl	Chlorpheniramine	8
	Phenylephrine	20
	Methscopolamine	2.5
Naldecon	Chlorpheniramine	5
	Phenyltoloxamine	15
	Phenylephrine	10
	Phenylpropanolamine	40
Novafed-A	Pseudoephedrine	120
	Chlorpheniramine	8
Ornade	Chlorpheniramine	8
	Phenylpropanolamine	50
	Isopropamide Iodide	2.5
Triaminic	Phenylpropanolamine	50
	Pheniramine	25
	Pyrilamine	25

* Where both capsule and tablet available only contents
  of capsule given

OTITIS MEDIA

INTRODUCTION

The term, "otitis," is often bandied about with gay abandon by various medical specialists; yet they frequently possess an imprecise conception of what this term really means or implies. "Otitis" simply means an inflammatory condition of the ear. However, without the appropriate modifiers, the term conveys very little information depicting the pathological processes involved or the implications for therapy. Otitis "media" designates the middle ear as the site of involvement. Table 1 provides a summary of the various types of disease processes which are labeled as otitis.

MECHANICAL OTITIS MEDIA

Serous Otitis Media

Mechanically induced otitis media, of which serous otitis provides a common example, results from Eustachian tube malfunction. Although some authorities theorize about the implications of viruses in the middle ear and immunological reactions of the middle ear mucosa, most agree that the principal etiologic factor is failure of middle ear aeration. In the resting state, the Eustachian tube orifice in the nasopharynx is closed. During the act of swallowing, the palatal muscles, principally the tensor veli palatini, levator veli palatini, and salpingopharyngeus, pull on the torus tubarius at the nasopharyngeal end of the tube causing it to open. Continuity is established between the middle ear cleft and the nasopharynx for about 600 msec which allows the free passage of air between the two. If the tubal orifice fails to open,

Figure 1:   ANATOMY OF THE EUSTACIAN TUBE

Schema showing the position of the levator muscle (1) with respect to the eustachian tube, superior tubal ligament (5) and two components of the tensor veli palatini muscle, one which tenses the palate (2) and the other which pulls the hook of the eustachian cartilage downward (3). Superior pharyngeal constrictor muscle (4).

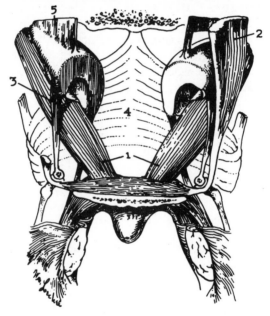

TABLE 1
Otitis Media

A. Mechanical
    1. Serous Otitis Media
        -- Acute
        -- Chronic
    2. Secretory Otitis Media ("Glue Ear")
    3. "Blue Ear"
B. Suppurative
    1. Acute Suppurative Otitis Media
    2. Chronic Suppurative Otitis Media
        (a) With Cholesteatoma   } (a) Active
        (b) Without cholesteatoma } (b) Quiescent
---

the air in the middle ear is absorbed by the rich net-
work of capillaries in the middle ear mucosa. As a
consequence, a negative pressure is set up that sucks
the tympanic membrane toward the promontory. The
negative pressure overcomes the oncotic pressure in
the capillaries, resulting in a transudation of yellow-
or amber-colored fluid into the middle ear space. This
so-called "serous otitis media" imposes a resistance
to the transmission of sound, producing a conductive
hearing loss.

Clinical Presentation

The patient suffering from this disorder is usually
a small child. Pain or even discomfort is an unusual
symptom. Often a pressure or fullness in the ears is
the complaint of older children. The commonest
symptom is hearing loss. This often goes unnoticed by
the child's parents although they report their child's
reluctance to come when called, turning up the audio
volume on the TV too high, or failure in school. These
all may be ascribed to diminished hearing acuity. In
toddlers, a tugging at the ears or unexplained
"fussiness" may be the only complaints.

Older children and adults suffering from this
malady may present with a history suggestive of baro-
trauma. A trip to the mountains during an upper
respiratory tract infection, scuba diving, or air
flight with Eustachian tube dysfunction are common

circumstances in this disorder. A nasopharyngeal mass
may obstruct the Eustacian tube orifice so that symptoms of denasal speech, nasal obstruction, and post-
nasal discharge must be carefully sought.
     Physical examination reveals a retracted tympanic
membrane with a dull cast to it. Amber fluid and
occasionally bubbles within it may be visualized in
the middle ear. The lack of mobility of the tympanic
membrane on pneumatic otoscopy is the key test that
makes the diagnosis. In the absence of an eardrum
perforation, this sign is pathognomonic of the presence
of middle ear fluid.
     Audiometric testing confirms a hearing loss of the
conductive type. A flat tympanometric curve indicates
an increased middle ear impedance resulting from the
presence of the middle ear effusion (Figure 2,3).

Etiology of Serous Otitis Media

     The causes of Eustachian tube dysfunction are
legion. The vast majority of the sufferers of acute
and chronic serous otitis media are small children,
and in many of these the precise etiology is uncertain.
A few of them have large adenoids that obstruct the
tubal orifice, and a few others have a chronic nasopharyngitis. Some children harbor bacteria and
purulent debris in the depths of the clefts in their
adenoid tissue. This causes edema of the adjacent
mucosa of the torus tubarius, resulting in difficulty
in tubal opening. However, the morbid role previously
assigned to the adenoids and tonsils as the principal
culprit in the genesis of Eustachian tube dysfunction
seems unjustified.
     The role of allergy has been implicated by many in
the past. There is no doubt that hypersensitivity
plays a part in a certain number of patients. The
finding of elevated immunoglobulins in middle ear
transudates has been reported by a number of investigators. However, in most studies, IgM and IgG levels
were equal to serum levels, and only IgA was elevated.
There was no evidence of elevated IgE levels in any
of the serous effusions. A positive family history or
suggestive association between symptomatology and

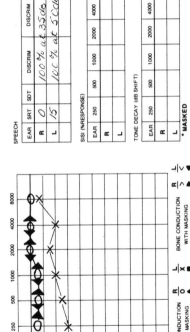

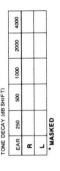

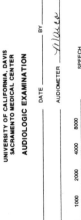

Figure 2: Audiogram illustrating the discrepancy between air conduction and bone conduction in the left ear compared to the normal right ear.

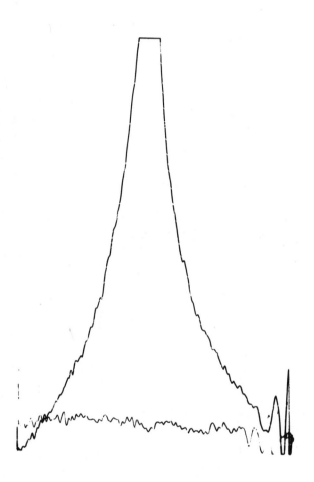

Figure 3: Tympanogram showing a normal curve in the right ear and a flat curve in the left ear indicating an increased impedance due to the presence of middle ear fluid.

potential inhalant or food allergens must be meticulously sought out. The principal reason for children to
develop serous effusions still remains an enigma.
"Eustacian tube immaturity" is more of an excuse for
ignorance than an explanation of the etiology in these
cases. In the young, the tube lies in a more horizontal plane than in the adult, and the lining mucosa
is thicker. Adenoids are more prominent, and lymphoid
tissue in general is more abundant. In mild defense
of this theory, it is surprising how most children,
as they progress toward puberty, outgrow their tendency
to develop serous otitis.
     When an adult presents with a unilateral serous
otitis, it is mandatory to examine the nasopharynx to
rule out nasopharyngeal carcinoma. Most cases of
serous otitis in adults are caused by acute upper
respiratory tract disorders often accompanied by baro-
trauma. However, if the condition does not clear after
a couple of weeks have passed, a nasopharyngeal tumor
must be excluded as the cause.
     Any condition affecting the palatal muscles that
control the Eustachian tubal orifice can result in
serous otitis. Individuals who suffer from cleft
palate have this as a common concomitant. Patients
suffering from palatal paralysis resulting from such
conditions as cerebral trauma, neuromuscular disease,
and Guillain-Barre syndrome will often have diminished
hearing because of serous otitis. Occasionally serous
otitis will be seen as the residuum of acute suppurative otitis media once the acute suppurative phase has
resolved. The residual fluid will be a sterile exudate
and differs pathophysiologically and biochemically from
the serous otitis that results from mechanical middle
ear disease.

Secretory Otitis Media

     Secretory otitis media differs from the serous
variety in a number of ways. This disorder is always
a chronic condition. The fluid is exceedingly thick
and viscid, henceits eponym "glue ear." The color is
clear or amber and may be translucent or opaque.
Secretory otitis is occasionally referred to as mucoid

otitis media, and this helps somewhat to explain its
genesis. The same etiological factors affecting the
Eustacian tube opening mechanism in serous otitis are
operative in this disease. The difference is that,
under the influence of chronic negative pressure, there
is a metaplasia of the middle ear mucosa with increases
in mucous glands and goblet cells. An outpouring of
mucous ensues and forms the "glue ear."

Clinical Presentation

The symptomatology of secretory otitis media is
eminently similar to serous otitis. The hearing loss
is often more profound because the mucoid fluid impedes
the motion of the ossicles to a greater extent than the
thinner serous fluid. Whereas a 15dB increase in
threshold is the usual sort of hearing loss seen in
serous otitis, losses of 30 and 45 dB are not uncommon
with secretory disease. On examination of the ears,
the tympanic membrane usually has a dull, slightly
bluish cast to it. Air bubbles are not seen. During
the negative pressure phase of pneumatic otoscopy, the
drumhead is often seen to wrinkle slightly, but is
essentially immobile.

Etiology of Secretory Otitis Media

The etiologic factors involved in secretory otitis
are again very similar to those involved in the production of chronic serous otitis media. One of the
notable exceptions is that there is much more definitive
evidence of the role of allergy in this disorder.
Reisman and Bernstein found, in an unselected group of
200 children with secretory otitis, a 23 percent
incidence of atopic disease. The incidence of allergy
in those that required multiple intubations of the
tympanic membrane for control of the disease was 35 percent. However, elevated IgE levels were not found in
the mucoid secretions in the middle ear with the
exception of two cases. It appears more likely that
the disease is the effect of the atopic process in the
nasopharynx rather than a direct effect on the middle
ear mucosa.

"Blue Ear"

This condition takes two forms. The first is merely
a variant of secretory otitis media. The blue cast it
gives the tympanic membrane is due to the breakdown
products of hemoglobin. Small hemorrhages occur in
the middle ear presumably secondary to the chronic
negative pressure that exists therein. The fluid in
"blue ear" contains broken down red blood cells and
cholesterin crystals. The second variety is due to
the presence of frank blood in the middle ear. Epistaxis that requires nasal packing produces this as
does the hemotympanum produced by a temporal bone
fracture. Occasionally a glomus jugulare tumor or a
high jugular bulb will impart a blue color to part of
the tympanic membrane. However, the findings of hearing loss and reduced drum mobility found in true "blue
ear" will not be present.

Treatment of Mechanical Otitis Media

The treatment essentially takes two forms: one, a
primary attack on the etiologic factors interfering
with Eustachian tube function and, the other, the
establishment of normal middle ear pressure and ablation
of the conductive hearing loss. In acute serous otitis
media, the basic pathological processes usually include
an involvement of the nasopharynx with an inflammatory
disease. Elimination of bacterial nasopharyngitis by
appropriate antibiotic therapy when a suppurative
process exists as well as treatment with an antihistaminic decongestant combination are the bulwarks of
therapy. When a viral process is responsible for the
problem, no antibiotics are indicated, and the antihistaminic decongestant combination will usually give
relief. Once the acute process is past, most adults
have spontaneous restoration of Eustachian tube
function and resolution of the serous otitis. If the
otitis persists, forced ventilation is performed with
a Politzer bag and/or in combination with the regular
practice by the patient of the modified Valsalva
maneuver. A few adult patients go on to develop chronic
serous otitis, and very few develop secretory otitis.

Acute serous otitis in children commonly accompanies an upper respiratory infection and frequently resolves spontaneously. However, in many the fluid persists to become chronic serous otitis. Once the nasopharynx and nose are free of infection, in addition to the medication, autoinflation of the Eustachian tube is attempted. Small children find the modified Valsalva maneuver difficult to perform. In lieu of this, the parents are encouraged to have their child autoinflate using "nose balloons." This contraption is simply constructed by tightly tying a worn, lax, toy rubber balloon to a nozzle. The nozzle is then inserted into the narés, and the child is instructed to inflate the balloon by blowing air through his nose through the nozzle while the contralateral naris is pinched shut. As the pressure in the balloon rises, the pressure at the nasopharyngeal end of the Eustachian tube does not   rise   until the seal is broken and air passes into the middle ear cleft.

Unfortunately, many children go on to develop chronic serous or secretory otitis media. If an allergic diathesis can be substantiated by sensitivity testing, desensitization may be successful in eliminating the effusion. Repair of a cleft palate is occasionally followed by resolution of the middle ear problem, but more often than not the effusion persists. The commonest correctable factor in the nasopharynx is the elimination of obstructive or chronically infected adenoids. Recurrent acute tonsillitis, without a concomitant adenoid infection or hypertrophy, will not in itself cause chronic mechanical otitis media. Adenoid infection is suggested by complaints of continuous purulent rhinorrhea and postnasal discharge. Obstructive adenoids make mouth breathing the rule and snoring at night a common complaint. Class II malocclusion, diastemata between the teeth, and retrognathia, the old stigmata of adenoid facies, are probably more myth than fact. However, the open mouth appearance of a child with obstructive adenoids does lend some credence to this notion. When obstructive or chronically infected adenoids are present with chronic secretory or serous otitis, adenoidectomy and myringotomy are advised. The provision of an alternative means of ventilating the middle ear was first introduced by Armstrong in 1954.

The ventilating tube does not cure chronic serous
or secretory otitis media, it merely obviates it until
the tube becomes plugged or extruded or the primary
problem responsible for Eustachian tube dysfunction is
resolved. If the patient avoids contamination of the
middle ear with water, the conductive hearing loss is
eliminated and he remains relatively free of middle ear
infections.

SUPPURATIVE OTITIS MEDIA

Suppurative otitis media is a bacterial infection
of the middle ear. It may be acute or chronic in
nature. Since the advent of antibiotics, the dangerous
sequelae of acute suppurative otitis media are uncommon.
Chronic suppurative otitis media that frequently
follows a poorly resolved acute suppurative episode is
similarly less common but, because of its indolent
nature presents more often with complications than the
acute suppurative variety.

Acute Suppurative Otitis Media

This disease entity is one of the commonest bacterial infections faced by the primary care physician. It
may appear de novo or result from secondary infection
of a preexistent middle ear effusion. The portal of
entry of the infecting organism is often the Eustachian
tube. A perforation of the tympanic membrane or a
tympanostomy tube can also provide access from the
external auditory canal. Bloodborne infections are
less common. The infecting organisms are commonly
Diplococcu pneumoniae, Streptococcus beta-hemolyticus,
Haemophilus influenzae, and rarely Staphylococcus
aureus.

Clinical Presentation

An upper respiratory tract infection usually precedes the illness. The patient suffers from malaise
and lethargy and becomes febrile and often toxic.
There is almost always otalgia and hearing loss. If
prompt antibiotic treatment is not administered, the

patient commonly has a spontaneous tympanic membrane
perforation, resulting in purulent drainage and
defervescence.

The disease actually progresses through a series
of stages. Although they form a continuum, specific
signs and symptoms characterize each stage and mandate
definite therapeutic steps. From the onset of the
disease, an untreated patient will progress through
the stages of hyperemia, exudation, and suppuration.
The course of the disease will culminate in either
stages of resolution or of coalescence and eventual
complication.

   a.   Stage of Hyperemia

      The patient is mildly febrile, suffers from
malaise, and feels lethargic. There is pain in the
ear (otalgia) and a feeling of fullness. Physical
examination reveals a mildly erythemic tympanic
membrane with dilated blood vessels around the anulus
and down the handle of the malleus. The membrane is
mobile on pneumatic otoscopy, unless there is a co-
existent serous or secretory otitis media. Hearing
is either normal or mildly depressed.

   b.   Stage of Exudation

      The fever increases, and, if the patient is a
child, convulsions may occur. Toxicity and prostration
are common. The otalgia increases in intensity, and
the hearing loss progresses. The tympanic membrane
bulges and is immobile. As this stage progresses, the
squamous epithelium over the drumhead begins to slough.
The middle ear is full of turbid, purulent fluid.
Ossicular landmarks, obvious in the hyperemic stage, are
now obscure.

   c.   Stage of Suppuration

      The tympanic membrane bursts, and a bloody,
purulent otorrhea drains through the perforation. The
patient defervesces, feels constitutionally better,
but the hearing loss persists. If the perforation
seals and pus reaccumulates, the symptoms of the stage

of hyperemia return and the drum reperforates. On
examination a ragged rent in the tympanic membrane is
apparent, exuding purulent, bloody fluid.
The fluid is often seen to pulsate. Once the pus is
cleansed from the canal, negative pressure is applied
with the pneumatic otoscope. If pus can be sucked
through the perforation in this way, this is called a
positive "reservoir sign." It is pathognomonic of
continued active disease and mandates vigorous treatment.

d. Stage of Resolution

        Upon rupture of the tympanic membrane and
drainage of pus, most cases of acute suppurative otitis
media resolve. The tympanic membrane seals within one
to three days, and the patient recovers. Occasionally
the perforation does not close, resulting in a chronic
suppurative otitis media. If this dehiscence is
adjacent to or involves the tympanic anulus, squamous
epithelium may grow into the middle ear, a condition
called cholesteatoma. Hearing in the resolved cases
usually returns to normal. If, however, ossicular
dissolution by pus should occur, it will result in a
residual hearing loss. The tympanic membrane may be
scarred, a condition called tympanosclerosis, and
fibrous tissue adhesions between the ossicles impeding
the normal movement may also be residua causing hearing
impairment.

Stage of Coalescence

    As has been stated, most untreated cases of this
disease resolve, but those that do not may progress
into the stage of coalescence. This is the starting
point of many severe, even life-threatening conditions.
During the stage of exudation, pus not only fills the
middle ear but the mastoid air cell system as well.
Some patients at this stage even show evidence of
erythema over the premastoid skin in the retroauricular
area. If the pus is allowed to remain, it slowly
causes decalcification of the thin bone comprising the
mastoid air cells. As this process nears completion
(taking, usually, from ten to fourteen days), it becomes

a coalescent mastoiditis. In the preantibiotic era,
this was a dreaded consequence of acute suppurative
disease as it often heralded many dire complications.

Coaslescent mastoiditis is characterized by a
swinging indolent fever, dull earache, hearing loss,
otorrhea, and anemia. The physical examination usually
reveals a chronically ill, pale, febrile individual
demonstrating erythema and often pitting edema of the
skin over the mastoid tip. There is usually chronic
otorrhea through a tympanic membrane perforation. A
sagging of the superior aspect of the external auditory
canal wall is frequently seen due to the subperiosteal
tracking of pus. The hearing is depressed. Mastoid
x-rays reveal a cloudiness to the mastoid air cell
system with loss of definition of the bony septa of
individual cells. The projection that most definitive-
ly contrasts this "ground glass" appearance of the
coalescent mastoid with the normal side on the same
film is the modified Towne view.

Stage of Complication

Improperly or untreated coalescent mastoiditis can
lead to numerous serious complications. Unfortunately,
limitations of space do not allow a complete dissert-
ation on them. The infection can break through the
mastoid cortex and present as a postauricular subperiosteal abscess, a zygomatic root abscess--just in
front of the ear--or even an abscess in the neck
(Bezold's abscess) that has tracked along the internal
jugular vein to present deep to the sternocleidomastoid.
Extension of disease into the organs contained within
the temporal bone may cause facial nerve paralysis,
vertigo, or sudden deafness. Progression of the
infection intracranially can result in meningitis,
temporal lobe or cerebellar cerebritis, perisinus
abscess, and brain abscess. Involvement of the dural
sinuses can cause thrombosis of the lateral or cavernous
sinuses. Involvement of the petrous apex in the
suppurative process can result in the symptoms of
Gradenigo's syndrome, consisting of pain behind the
ear on the affected side (from involvement of the
ophthalmic branch of the fifth cranial nerve), a lateral
rectus palsy (resulting from a sixth nerve neuritis),

and a draining ear.

Treatment of Acute Suppurative Otitis Media

Early and appropriate treatment is absolutely
essential in order to avoid the many disastrous
complications that are possible from acute suppurative
otitis media. In most practices, the majority of
patients are seen during the stage of hyperemia. The
implementation of the appropriate antibiotic therapy,
such as ampicillin for those under age six and penicillin
for the majority of the remaining patients, should be
given in full therapeutic doses. The addition of an
antihistaminic-decongestant combination helps to reduce
edema and swelling in the nasopharynx which predispose
the patient to this otologic disease. Bed rest, fluids
by mouth, and systemic analgesics are given. Most
analgesic ear drops should be avoided. The basic
ingredient in many of them is phenol which causes
destruction of the squamous layer of the tympanic
membrane. If the patient has progressed to the stage
of exudation and the drum is bulging, a myringotomy
should be done. A myringotomy is preferred over
spontaneous rupture because the site of the perforation
can be planned in order to avoid the so-called marginal
perforation (one that occurs adjacent to the tympanic
anulus) that may occur from rupture of the tympanic
membrane. After the tympanic membrane incision has been
made, the myringtomy knife is run along an agar plate
for culture. The myringotomy should be repeated every
day until pus stops draining. If the patient is not
seen until after a spontaneous rupture has occurred,
then the drainage is cultured and the antibiotic and
antihistaminic-decongestant combination are employed.
Antibiotic-steroid combination ear drops are of marginal
value in an acutely suppurating ear. The drops are
quicklydiluted, thus neutralized by the pus, and have
little chance of making contact with the underlying
mucosa or bone. It is important to follow the patient
once the acute process has subsided to ascertain that
the perforation will close spontaneously. If it does
not, surgical intervention should be entertained.
Coalescent mastoiditis was once entirely a

surgical disease. Since the advent of antibiotics, it
is an uncommon disease. In its early stages, the
process can still be reversed by intensive antibiotic
therapy, however, in many cases no subsequent resolution ensues and mastoidectomy is indicated. Once the
mastoiditis progresses to the stage of complication,
vigorous antibiotic therapy, followed within twelve
to twenty-four hours or even less by mastoidectomy, is
many times life saving.

Chronic Suppurative Otitis Media

Any ear with a hole in the tympanic membrane is
described as having chronic suppurative otitis media.
In that most perforations result from an acute
suppurative otitis media, this is a valid concept.
However, there are some perforations that are secondary
to trauma. Those that stay open may be due to a
secondary infection that occurred some time in the
course of the disease. However, it is unlikely that
this applies to most traumatic perforations that
persist. Here the definition does somewhat break down.
The disease can be either active or quiescent.
When there is frank, manifest suppuration, the disease
is described as active. The pus is usually thick and
green. The principal infecting organism is Pseudomonas
species, which is a common inhabitant of the external
auditory canal. The perforation can be either central
or marginal. Marginal ones involve the tympanic anulus
and permit free access for migration of external
auditory canal skin into the middle ear. The incidence
of squamous epithelial migration into the middle ear is
only 10 percent for central perforations but 85 percent
for those of the marginal variety. Chronic suppurative
otitis media may be accompanied by cholesteatoma.

Clinical Presentation

The symptoms of chronic suppurative otitis media
are often occult. Hearing loss is a common complaint
and may be longstanding and not noticed much by the
patient. Periodic suppuration is also common, and
the physician must be alert in questioning the patient
as to frequency of occurrence, volume, color, consist-

ency, and odor of the drainage. The frequency, amount, duration, and responsiveness to therapy are often an indicator of the severity of this disease. The color and odor may give clues to the underlying cause of the otorrhea. For example, a thin, watery, highly foul smelling drainage is characteristic of osteomyelitis of the temporal bone, whereas a thick, greenish, musty smelling drainage is common with cholesteatoma infected with Pseudomonas. It is important to know if there is a past history of a seventh-nerve paralysis or vertigo. Cholesteatoma can invade the Fallopian canal of the facial nerve as well as erode the bone of the horizontal semicircular canal of the labyrinth. Pain is rather uncommon except occasionally just preceding the onset of the drainage. If a painful otorrhea persists despite vigorous local treatment, a high index of suspicion for carcinoma of the external ear canal or middle ear should be maintained.

Chronic suppurative otitis is commonly a long-standing problem often originating in childhood. The problem of inadequate Eustachian tube function, that so often plagues the pediatric age group, is again the culprit in this disease. One of the problems of re-habilitating individuals with this disease is restoration of tubal function. Oftentimes what began in childhood as a problem at the nasopharyngeal end with interference of tubal opening becomes in later life a problem of tubal patency in the middle ear. This end becomes obstructed with granulation tissue, polypoid mucosa, and purulent debris.

Physical examination usually confirms the presence of a hearing loss. Very commonly the loss is mixed, with the anticipated conductive component secondary to disruption of the middle ear and the sensorineural component secondary to possibly a toxic effect of the chronic infectious process on the inner ear. The loss may be profound and may be extremely debilitating.

The perforation is seen on inspection of the tympanic membrane but may be obscured by pus if the disease is active. Silver flakes of desquamated skin, if seen floating in the pus, are highly suspicious signs of cholesteatoma. The pus and debris must be adequately cleansed by gentle suction followed by wiping

78

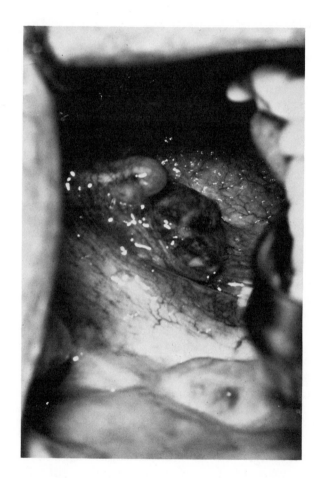

Figure 4: View of oropharynx illustrating a prolapsing lymphoepithelioma of nasopharynx.

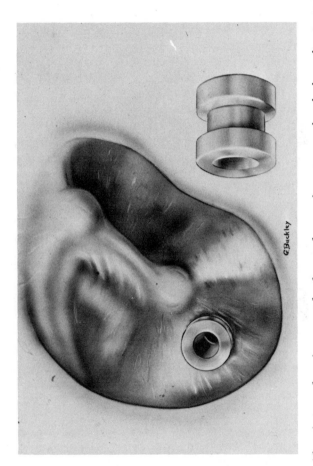

Figure 5: Ventilating tube inserted through myringotomy incision in tympanic membrane.

with small cotton swabs. A positive reservoir sign and
pulsation of the purulent exudate indicate the severity
of the active process. Pneumatic otoscopy must be
performed to not only look for the reservoir sign but
also to look for the presence of the "fistula sign."
If on positive pressure, the eyes deviate to the
opposite side, followed by a few quick beats of nystagmus, this is a positive fistula test. This indicates
that the disease process has eroded the bone of the
horizontal semicircular canal down to the endosteum.
Pressure exerted by air from the pneumatic otoscope
through the tympanic membrane perforation against the
endosteum pushes a wave of perilymph in the horizontal
semicircular canal which causes a secondary wave in
the endolymph of the corresponding semicircular duct.
The wave in the duct pushes against the cupula, driving
it toward the utricle, setting in motion the ocular
reflex that results in nystagmus. This sign indicates
that the ear is in danger of developing the complication of suppurative labyrinthitis. Occasionally the
external auditory canal will be filled with a mucosal
polyp. This should be removed only by an otologist
because of the inherent danger of snatching the
ossicles.

Treatment of Chronic Suppurative Otitis

Management of these disorders involves both medical
and surgical modalities. If the ear is actively
suppurating, often a thorough evaluation of the extent
of disease is impossible. After thorough mechanical
cleansing, the patient is placed on a regimen of saline
or dilute vinegar ear washes four times daily. One
quart of sterile saline or one-fourth strength household vinegar is lavaged through the ear with a soft
rubber bulb syringe at each session. Following this,
four drops of antibiotic-steroid combination ear drops
are placed in the affected ear. Unless signs of
systemic illness are present, which is most rare unless
a complication is present, systemic antibiotics are of
little value. The irrigations and drops are continued
for ten to twenty-one days then followed for one week
by drops only. The ear is then reassessed. If the

perforation becomes dry and Eustachian tube patency can be established by the passage of air, then a simple patching of the ear drum (myringoplasty) is sufficient treatment. If, however, the ear continues to suppurate, a mastoidectomy will be required to eradicate the disease. When cholesteatoma is present, mastoidectomy is almost always indicated. If the patient presents with a complication, immediate surgical intervention is required once antibiotic therapy has been instituted.

REFERENCES

Mogi G, Honjo S, Maeda S, Yoshida T: Secretory immuno-globulin A(SIgA) in middle ear effusions. Ann Otol Rhinol Laryngol 82: 302-310, 1973.

Veltri RW, Sprinkle PM: Serous otitis media: Immuno-globulin and lysozyme levels in middle ear fluids and serum. Ann Otol Rhinol Laryngol 82: 297-301, 1973.

Tonder O, Gundersen T: Nature of the fluid in serous otitis media. Arch Otolaryngol 93: 473-478, 1971.

Mogi G, Maeda S, Yoshida T, Watanabe N: Otitis media with effusion: Specific antibody activities against exotoxins in middle ear effusions. Laryngoscope 86: 1043-1055, 1976.

Clemis J: Allergic tubotympanitis. Otolaryngol Clin North Am 4(3): 549-555, 1971.

Reisman RE, Bernstein J: Allergy and secretory otitis media. Pediatr Clin North Am 22(1): 251-257, 1975.

Wiederhold ML, Zajtchuk JT, Vop JG, de Fries HO: Viscosity characteristics of middle ear effusions. Surg Forum 29: 587-588, 1978.

Armstrong B: A new treatment for chronic secretory otitis media. Arch Otolaryngol 59: 653-654, 1954.

Donald PJ, McCabe BF, Loevy S: Atticotomy: A neglected otosurgical technique. Ann Otol Rhinol Laryngol 83: 652-663, 1974.

Paparella MM, Makato O, Hiraide F, Brady D: Pathology of sensorineural hearing loss in otitis media. Ann Otol Rhinol Laryngol 81: 632-647, 1972.

Michael H. Keslin

EVALUATION AND CHARACTERIZATION
OF ASTHMA

INTRODUCTION

Asthma lacks a crisp definition because it is a heterogeneous disorder with a wide constellation of clinical associations, all having in common the final denominator of bronchospasm. Classically, it has been characterized by wheezing, dyspnea and severe chest congestion, but this probably represents only the severe end of a spectrum. Indeed in many, the only complaints are a cough or even chronic congestion of the throat mistakenly attributed to post-nasal drainage. Thus, the well known musical rales are frequently absent; almost all patients demonstrate mild to severe reversible increases in airway resistance.

PREVALENCE OF ASTHMA

Asthma accounted for 1,795,000 private patient visits during 1975; 44% of these patients were seen by allergists, 32% by family practitioners, 10% by internists and 8% by pediatricians. 52% of the patients were male and 48% female. Over 90% of these patients required some form of drug therapy. The mortality of asthma is low, but nonetheless, it may account for up to 2,000 deaths per year, and the majority of these fatalities occur in children. In fact, asthma is the most common chronic disease of childhood. However, although the mortality of asthma is low, the morbidity is significant. Approximately 150,000 hospital admissions a year result from asthma. In addition, the unpredictable nature of asthma can have a devastating effect on the psychological well-being of the patient and family. The chronic and physically restricting nature of the disease often results in anger, frustration, depression and anxiety.

These emotional responses often make the asthma itself
worse and, therefore, make the disease more difficult to
manage.

HETEROGENEITY OF ASTHMA

The classification of this disorder has always been
arbitrary and none has ever been totally satisfactory.
Table 1 outlines four major variables, 1) factors that
precipitate attacks, 2) predisposing constitutional factors, 3) bronchial response patterns, and 4) response to
therapeutic agents. This represents a more practical
clinical and therapeutic approach as opposed to those
based on biochemical and physiologic parameters.

TABLE 1

How Asthmatics Vary
1. Factors that precipitate attacks
    A. Allergens
    B. ASA and nonsteroidal anti-inflammatory drugs
    C. Tartrazine
    D. Viral respiratory tract infections
    E. Irritants
    F. Exercise
    G. Situations and emotional responses
2. Predisposing constitutional factors
    A. Immunologic status
        1. IgE response
        2. IgA deficient
    B. Irritability of airways
    C. Endocrine status
3. Bronchial Response Patterns
    A. Location of airway obstruction
    B. Tempo of obstruction
    C. Smooth muscle spasm
    D. Bronchial inflammation
    E. Mucous glands
    F. Degree of reversibility
4. Response to Therapeutic Agents
    A. Theophylline metabolism (see page 101)
    B. Cromolyn sodium
    C. "Paradoxical" response to Isoproterenol
    D. Troleandomycin

FACTORS THAT PRECIPITATE ATTACKS

A. Allergens

Approximately 40 to 50% of asthmatics have elevated
levels of IgE to specific antigens, i.e., pollens, house
dust, mold spores, animal danders, and foods. These are
detected by appropriate skin testing techniques or RAST.
Inhalation of these antigens in a sensitized patient may
trigger bronchospasm, presumably by a mechanism that
involves combination of antigen with cell-fixed antigen-
specific IgE resulting in the release of various pharmacological mediators such as histamine and slow reacting
substance of anaphylaxis. Many inhalants, such as
pollen grains, are too large to penetrate deeply into
the lungs. Patterson et al. recently demonstrated that
respiratory lumen cells may transfer bronchial reactivity for a specific antigen from sensitized to non-re-
active rhesus monkeys. Since these are the first cells
exposed to inhaled antigens, they propose these cells
may play a major role in initiating the IgE mediated
airway response by releasing vasoactive mediators and
potentiating the penetration of inhaled antigens into
deeper tissues of the respiratory tract, thereby ampli-
fying the allergic response.
Foods are not commonly known as inhalants, however,
specific occupational exposures to grains and aerosolized fish lead to job related but readily treatable
asthma in bakers and food processors. Asthma may also
be produced by the ingestion of foods. If the reaction
is immediate, there are usually significant detectable
levels of IgE antibody to the specific food. Unfortunately, this is an unusual manifestation and the routine
use of food skin testing in chronic asthmatics is probably valueless.

B. Aspirin and Non-steroidal Anti-inflammatory Drugs

Approximately 2% to 4% of asthmatic patients give a
history of asthma attacks precipitated by aspirin ingestion. However, 15% to 20% of asthmatics may have
evidence of significant obstructive airway disease
demonstrated after challenge with aspirin. These challenge studies are usually done with an initial dose of

15-35 mgs. of acetylsalicylic acid and thence sequentially increasing the dose on subsequent days until the
patient develops a 20% fall in his forced expiratory
volume in one second, or until he has taken a dose equi-
valent to 600 mgs. of aspirin. Using this protocol,
under carefully controlled conditions, aspirin challenge
studies are relatively safe. There have been reports,
however, of fatalities in patients suspected of being
aspirin intolerant, who were given therapeutic doses of
aspirin as a means of determining aspirin intolerance.
Moreover, some patients who are intolerant to aspirin
may also be intolerant to nonsteroidal anti-inflammatory
drugs such as indomethacin or mefenamic acid, although
most of these patients can tolerate sodium salicylate.
Rare patients have been described who are intolerant to
acetaminophen. Patients who are aspirin intolerant
frequently also have evidence of chronic sinus disease
and nasal polyposis (see page 235).

C. Tartrazine Dye

    Approximately one third of aspirin intolerant asth-
matics develop asthma after ingesting as little as 1 mg.
of tartrazine dye. However, almost all patients who are
tartrazine intolerant are also aspirin intolerant. This
yellow azobenzene dye, classified as FD&C #5, is a ubiquitous coloring agent in multiple foods and drugs (see
Chapter 7). Patients who are tartrazine intolerant must
meticulously regulate their diet to avoid this substance.
Tartrazine challenge tests are often helpful and do not
seem to be fraught with the same dangers as aspirin
challenge.

D. Viral Respiratory Tract Infections

    Viruses likely to trigger asthma in small children
include respiratory syncytial virus (RSV) and parain-
fluenza virus (PV). In older children and adults,
rhinovirus and influenza virus are much more common.
Many patients associate their first episode of asthma
with a viral infection with RSV, myxovirus or mycoplasma
and the asthmatic state persists after the infection has
subsided. Epithelial damage may stimulate the afferent
limb of the vagal reflex resulting in reflex broncho-

constriction through afferent vagal discharge, or a
product of the virus infected cell might interfere with
beta adrenergic responses and make bronchial cells hy-
perreactive to cholinergic or perhaps alpha adrenergic
stimuli. These hypotheses, however, are not well substantiated. Moreover, immunization with such agents has
had significant adverse effects in asthmatic children.

E. Irritants

Various non-specific stimuli such as cold air, air
pollution, cigarette smoke, perfumes, insecticides and
some petrochemicals may trigger episodes of asthma.
Increased amounts of "smog" affect not only asthmatics
but almost all patients with chronic obstructive lung
disease. Oxides of sulfur, sulfuric acid and particulate matter are common in large cities (i.e. London) and
result from the combustion of fossil fuels; whereas
ozones, nitrogen oxides and hydrocarbons predominate in
sunny, warm climates (i.e. Los Angeles), because of the
heavy automobile traffic and photochemical processes.
Toulene diisocyanate (TDI), a catalyst used in the production of polyurethane foam, has been associated with
severe episodes of bronchospasm in asthmatic patients,
even in concentrations of less than 0.02 parts per
million.

F. Exercise

Although exercise often precipitates bronchospasm
in the chronic asthmatic patient, there is a subsection
of asthmatics in whom the attack is brought on only by
exercise. The type of exercise is important. Free
range running commonly induces asthma, whereas swim-
ming produces almost no symptoms. Strauss et al. have
recently demonstrated that the critical factors may well
be the adverse effects of low temperature and low humidity of inspired air.

G. Emotional Responses

Patients with asthma are frequently hostile and depressed. These are probably emotional responses to the
disease rather than specific personality types.

Although emotional upsets may occasionally trigger
attacks,   routine psychiatric evaluation seems
unwarranted.

PREDISPOSING CONSTITUTIONAL FACTORS

    The ability to form elevated levels of IgE in re-
sponse to antigen exposure through the respiratory and
gastrointestinal route is genetically determined and
euphemistically referred to as "atopic". In contrast,
congenital IgA deficiency which is frequently associated
with atopy, occurs in about one in five hundred births
and is the most frequent type of immunodeficiency.
Moreover, there is a strong familial incidence of IgA
deficiency and the incidence of IgE mediated disease
seems higher in IgA deficient patients. It should be
noted at least one third of asthmatics have episodes
primarily triggered by type I IgE mediated reactions.
The role of IgA is unclear. It is the principal antibody in the secretions of the respiratory and gastrointestinal tracts and it has, therefore, been speculated
that low levels may predispose to the development of
viral respiratory and/or gastrointestinal infections.
    All asthmatic patients studied to date have demon-
strated exquisite sensitivity to methacholine, a synthetic analogue of the cholinergic neural transmitter,
acetylcholine, and many patients are similarly sensitive
to low doses of inhaled histamine. Such abnormalities
suggest an imbalance in the autonomic nervous system
control of the airways, as manifest by heightened sensitivity to cholinergic and, perhaps, alpha adrenergic
stimuli and reduced sensitivity to beta adrenergic stimuli.
    Asthma usually increases in severity during hyper-
thyroidism. It is also very severe in adrenocortical
insufficiency. Altered corticosteroid metabolism is a
speculated but unproven mechanism in the above. In
contrast, pregnancy usually results in improvement of
asthma, although occasional patients note increased
difficulty. Finally, there are rare asthmatics whose
disease exacerbates during the menstrual cycle.

BRONCHIAL RESPONSE PATTERNS

Asthmatic patients demonstrate heterogeneity in the location of airway obstruction. Some have a rapid onset of bronchoconstriction followed by a relatively brisk response to therapy. Such patients usually demonstrate their obstruction primarily in larger central airways. In others, there is a gradual onset of bronchospasm over days and weeks; often associated with a longer recovery time. In the latter, the obstruction is primarily in the peripheral airways, with increased mucus production and associated airway plugging.

The obstructive phenomena seen in asthma is produced by varying degrees of bronchospasm and bronchial wall inflammation, resulting in partial obliteration of the lumen, and increased amounts of bronchial mucus. Smooth muscle spasm is most often seen following a discrete antigen challenge, i.e. animal dander in a sensitized patient. Bronchial inflammation is the significant factor in asthma associated with viral respiratory infections and exposure to toxic fumes; a late onset pattern with asthma developing 4 to 12 hours after exposure is common with the latter. Similarly, some patients seem prone to production of thick tenacious mucus during acute episodes. This is often associated with relatively severe asthma requiring corticosteroids. These patients are, in particular, candidates for status asthmaticus. Marked reversibility of airway obstruction is usually associated with primarily a bronchospastic component, whereas mucus plugging and bronchial inflammation predominate in those who have a persistent significant impairment in their expiratory flow rates.

LEVELS OF ASTHMA THERAPY

An understanding of the basic pathophysiology of asthma and sites of action of various drugs used in therapy is essential for a rational approach to the treatment of this disease. As we have previously noted, the underlying feature of asthma is the presence of hyper-reactive airways. With appropriate stimuli, these airways develop bronchospasm, mucosal edema and mucus plugging. This results in increased work of breathing, CO_2 retention and hypoxia which in turn causes increased

bronchospasm. Ventilation perfusion abnormalities also
develop which result in further hypoxia which in turn,
increases bronchospasm. Hypoxia and CO_2 retention
cause increased pulmonary resistance and pulmonary hypertension.

Asthma therapy occurs at four levels. The first
level involves out-patient management, the second speaks
to the assessment and management of acutely ill patients,
the third, management of status asthmaticus, and the
fourth, mechanical ventillation in those patients with
respiratory failure.

OUT-PATIENT MANAGEMENT OF ASTHMA

The first step in managing patients is to identify
the relevant precipitating and predisposing factors.
This involves careful history, physical examination and
frequently allergy skin tests. The second step is to
design an individualized therapeutic program for the
patient which provides optimal functional capacity with
minimal side effects. Most physicians feel that one
should either start with a theophylline preparation or
a selective Beta$_2$ adrenergic agonist. A number of oral
theophylline preparations are currently available.
These include Aminophyllin, which is approximately 83%
anhydrous theophylline and oxtriphylline (Choledyl),
which is approximately 64% anhydrous theophylline. The
dose of theophylline is approximately 4 mg/kg per dose,
although (please see p. 101), there is a wide patient
variation in serum half-lives. Most adults are begun
on a dose of 200 to 300 mgs. of Aminophyllin or Choledyl
four times a day. The dose can be adjusted upward or
downward depending upon clinical response and development of various side effects, such as, gastrointestinal
irritation, nausea, vomiting or diarrhea. Gastrointestinal side effects are minimized if the drug is given
with meals. Theophylline blood levels are helpful in
determining the correct dose in patients who seem to
develop side effects on low doses or in patients who
do not develop the anticipated response to the drug.
Blood levels can be obtained just prior to the next
scheduled dose. The usual therapeutic range is 10-20
mcg/ml. Side effects, such as nervousness, nausea,
vomiting, anorexia and headache have been found to

correlate with serum concentrations greater than 20 mcg/
ml. Seizures have been reported at serum concentrations
greater than 30 mcg/ml and cardiac arrhythmias are a
potential hazard with concentrations greater than 40
mcg/ml.

Sympathomimetic agents appear to potentiate beta receptor stimulation resulting in generation of increased
levels of intracellular cyclic AMP. Some result in
alpha adrenergic stimulation, generating increased
cyclic GMP and consequent bronchoconstriction. Ephedrine is the oral beta adrenergic agent usually found in
fixed-combination bronchodilators marketed in this
country. It is the least effective of this group of
drugs and has both alpha and beta activity. Studies
have demonstrated only equivocal improvement when added
to an adequate program of theophylline therapy; however,
it does significantly increase the incidence of side
effects, i.e. tremor and nervousness. The recent division of the beta receptor into Beta$_1$-adrenoceptors
and beta$_2$-adrenoceptors has led to marked changes in the
pharmacotherapy of asthma. Stimulation of beta$_1$ receptors results in increased heart rate, dilation of coronary blood vessels and relaxation of smooth muscle of
the gastrointestinal tract, whereas, specific stimulation of beta$_2$ receptors results in relaxation of the
smooth muscle of the bronchi. Terbutaline is an excellent oral beta$_2$ agonist; however, it may cause significant tremor which could limit optimal dosage. Metaproterenol has somewhat less beta$_2$ specificity, but is less
likely to cause tremor. Recently, Wolfe et al. demonstrated that 5 mgs. of terbutaline produced about the
same degree of bronchodilatation as 400 mgs of aminophylline in moderately severe asthmatics. The combination, however, of these two drugs in the same dosage
produced significantly greater bronchodilatation than
either drug alone. A combination of 2.5 mgs. of terbutaline and 200 mgs. of aminophylline produced bronchodilatation equal to the higher dose of either drug
alone. Low doses of both drugs, therefore, may be ad-
vantageous in patients who experience unacceptable side
effects from high doses of either drug. The usual
starting dose of terbutaline is 2.5 mgs. four times a
day or metaproterenol 10 mgs. four times a day.

Cromolyn sodium, another frequently used agent, is
not a bronchodilator, but is felt to block the release
of mediators from sensitized mast cells. This drug is
only effective in preventing episodes of asthma and has
no place in the treatment of acute episodes. It is administered by oral inhalation from a spinhaler which
aerosolyzes the powder in the capsule; usual dose is 20
mgs. four times a day and an adequate trial usually requires using the drug for two to four weeks. At that
time, a decision can be made as to whether or not the
drug should be continued. The drug has been particularly helpful in blocking exercise-induced asthma when it
is used 30 to 45 minutes prior to exercise. It has also
been found helpful in blocking asthma secondary to exposure to toluene diisocyanate. The side effects of
cromolyn include cough, transient bronchospasm, maculo-
papular rash, and four reported cases of pulmonary in-
filtrate with eosinophilia. The disadvantages of the
drug are poor patient compliance, because of the incon-
venient route of administration and relatively high
costs. A one month supply of the drug costs the patient
about $25.00 to $30.00. Use of this drug should be considered in any patient requiring long-term, relatively
high dose medication for control of his asthma; 60% to
75% of the patients will show a significant improvement
in their symptoms.

Beclomethasone diproprionate is a "non-absorbable"
inhaled steroid that has only recently been marketed in
the United States and has created a minor revolution in
the treatment of steroid dependent bronchial asthma.
In spite of the "non-absorbable" label, there is a demonstrable though minimal suppression of the pituitary-
adrenal axis that is dose related. Patients are usually
started on two sprays by inhalation four times a day and
maximized at four sprays four times per day. With an
appropriate response, oral steroids are gradually tapered, but are never abruptly discontinued. Serum corti-
sols will help determine if and the speed with which
this can be accomplished. The only major problem has
been pharyngeal candidiasis in approximately 5-10% of
the patients, and for this reason, it is suggested that
patients rinse and gargle thoroughly with clear water
after each usage to remove the steroid from the mouth
and pharynx. One episode of candidiasis should not

preclude future use. Oral glucocorticoids may be used
in short courses to treat acute exacerbations of asthma
particularly those associated with respiratory tract infections and acute antigen exposure. The dosage is usually 20 to 40 mgs. of prednisone twice a day for three
to five days and discontinued without tapering. Except
for occasional acute psychosis and mild salt retention,
there are no significant side effects. Patients with
more severe chronic asthma who are not effectively controlled on theophylline, beta adrenergic agents, and/or
beclomethasone and have had a trial of sodium cromolyn,
may require long-term steroid therapy. A short-acting
steroid, such as prednisone or methylprednisolone is
preferred, and, if possible, the drug given only in the
morning. This format, commonly known as "booster"
therapy, presumes that the drug functions additively
with the normal high A.M. cortisol. This allows for
normal adrenal stimulation once the drug is metabolized.
Every other day steroid therapy represents an even
further advance utilizing this hypothesis. It can dramatically reduce the side effects of Cushingoid facies,
weight gain, and striae. Patients who have been on
chronic daily steroids for years may have extremely
suppressed adrenal function and adrenal function should
be assessed before attempting this regimen.

Immunotherapy may be beneficial in treating patients
with IgE mediated bronchospasm. However, long-term well
controlled clinical trials have not been accomplished
to determine its efficacy. It is still the opinion of
many allergists that it is an effective treatment mo-
dality, particularly in pollen related asthma.

The cornerstone of successful out-patient management of asthma is patient education. This includes a
thorough explanation of the nature of the disease, the
relative etiologic factors in a given case, the mechanism of action of the various drugs used to treat the
disease and the potential side effects of these drugs.
Patients also need to be carefully advised how to modi-
fy their medications if their asthma is increasing and
whom to contact in emergency situations. Good patient
education results in decreased patient anxiety about
the disease, which in turn, facilitates successful management.

ASSESSMENT AND TREATMENT OF ACUTELY ILL PATIENTS

Factors which should alert the physician to the possibility that an acute attack of asthma is likely to require vigorous therapy in a given patient are a history
of previous severe attacks, hospitalization, and/or
requirement for use of large doses of corticosteroids.
Patients who develop acute asthmatic attacks while on
a previously optimal therapeutic program also need to
be observed carefully and followed closely. Physical
examination can be misleading in trying to assess the
severity of obstructive airway disease. Physical signs
found to be of value include the presence of a paradoxical pulse which suggests that the forced expiratory
volume in 1 second (FEV_1) is less than 1.25 L. Furthermore, retraction of sternocleidomastoid muscles suggests
that the FEV_1 is less than 1 L. and that there is a
high degree of airway resistance. Arterial blood gases
usually reveal moderate arterial hypoxemia (PaO_2 of 50
to 70 mm/Hg), hypocapnea and respiratory alkalosis. A
normal $PaCO_2$ in an acutely ill asthmatic is a serious
finding and may indicate impending respiratory failure.
The most direct way of assessing the severity of obstructive airway disease is to do simple pulmonary
function tests, such as, FEV_1, forced vital capacity
(FVC), or maximum midexpiratory flow rates (MMEF). FEV_1
and MMEF usually average only 30% or less of predicted
values during acute attacks of asthma. The FVC averages
50% of predicted. Electrocardiogram changes, such as,
right axis deviation, P-pulmonale, or right ventricular
hypertrophy indicate severe asthma. These changes are
often rapidly reversible with adequate therapy of the
obstructive airway disease. Chest x-ray is helpful in
looking for signs of pneumonia, atelectasis, pneumothorax or pneumomediastinum. Similarly, it has been
demonstrated that Emergency Room evaluation of patients
with acute asthma can be facilitated by monitoring the
improvement in FEV_1. They demonstrated that two-thirds
of the patients with less than a 400 ml increase in
FEV_1 may relapse and therefore require further out-
patient therapy or perhaps hospital admission. Only
29% of patients who demonstrated greater than 400 ml
improvement in FEV_1 following Emergency Room treatment,
suffered relapse and required further emergency

treatment or hospital admission.

The objectives of treatment of an acute episode of asthma are first of all, to produce significant improvement in bronchospasm. The second and equally important objective is to establish a good program of oral bronchodilator therapy and make arrangements for close outpatient followup with serial determinations of pulmonary function and clinical status. Antibiotics are indicated if bacterial infection or superimposed bacterial process is felt to be a factor in the acute attack. Oral steroids are indicated in moderate to severe episodes in patients who have previously been on optimal programs of oral theophylline or $beta_2$ stimulant drugs. In patients who are already on long-term steroid therapy, a three day steroid boost may be required. Usually, the maintenance dosage of prednisone is doubled and administered every eight to twelve hours for approximately 72 hours; often the patient can then be placed back on his maintenance steroid dose.

STATUS ASTHMATICUS

The protocol for management of status asthmaticus is outlined in Table 2. This is a life-threatening illness and the vast majority of deaths occur in this state. It is defined as severe asthma unresponsive to inhaled or injected sympathomemetic agents or maximum oral, or intravenous theophylline. Patients must be closely monitored and, again, a thorough search made for precipitating factors, i.e. infection, inhaled bronchodilator abuse, antigen exposure, cardiac failure, dehydration. Steroids should not be tapered at all until there is an obvious clinical response at which point one could switch to an oral preparation. In the vast majority, they will be discharged on a tapering dose.

RESPIRATORY FAILURE

Scoggin et al. recently reviewed their experience with 811 patients treated at the Colorado General Hospital for status asthmaticus over an eight year period between 1967 and 1975. Twenty-one of these patients required mechanical ventilation, and the overall

mortality in their hands was approximately 1%. Of the
twenty-one patients who required mechanical ventilation,
eight expired resulting in a mortality of 40% in this
group. A summary of the factors to be considered in
mechanical ventilation of patients with respiratory
failure secondary to asthma is outlined in Table 3.

TABLE 2

Management of Status Asthmaticus
A. Arterial blood gases (ABG) stat
B. O_2 by nasal cannula at 5 L/min.
C. Repeat ABG's in 20 min. and adjust $F_1 O_2$ as indicated.
   Rate of $PaCO_2$ increase is more important than actual
   amount of change.
D. IV fluids and potassium replacement--correct dehydration, but avoid over hydration.
E. IV aminophyllin
   1. Loading dose 5.6 mg/kg over 20 min. maintenance
      dose .9 mg/kg/hr.
   2. $T_{(1/2)}$ of theophyllin lengthened in old age, CHF
      or liver disease.
   3. Nomogram available for calculating loading and
      maintenance doses.
   4. Therapeutic range is 10 to 20 mg/L.
F. IV corticosteroids
   1. Studies of dose-response relationship in status
      asthmaticus not available.
   2. Usual doses employed.
      a) Methylprednisolone(Medrol) 40 mg every 4-6
         hrs.
      b) Hydrocortisone 200 mg. every 4-6 hrs.
   3. Doses in this range usually continued for 3-4
      days and then tapered as rapidly as clinical
      situation allows. Can switch to oral steroid
      (e.g. prednisone) in equivalent doses and con-
      tinue tapering on outpatient basis.
G. Maximist treatments (8 drops bronkosol in 4 cc. NaCl)
   followed by postural drainage and percussion every
   4-6 hrs.
H. Monitor pulmonary functions (FEV_1, MMEF) daily at
   bedside.

TABLE 3

1. Indications for mechanical ventilation
    A. Severe deterioration in mental status.
    B. Progressive increase in $PaCO_2$.
2. Principles for use of mechanical ventilation in status asthmaticus.
    A. Use large ET tube (8mm or larger) and insert by nasotracheal route, if possible.
    B. Use volume-cycled ventilator (TV=10 to 12 ml/kg).
    C. Humidification to facilitate removal of mucus.
    D. Use lowest possible cycling pressure that allows adequate alveolar ventilation.
    E. Keep respiratory rate as slow as possible (10-12 /min) to allow adequate time for expiratory phase--this will help to diminish further air trapping.
    F. Avoid hypocapnia which may potentiate arrhythmias, seizures, bronchospasm and reduced cardiac output.
    G. If suppression of respiratory drive necessary, avoid histamine releasing drugs such as morphine, meperidine, or succinylcholine, diazepam or pancuronium are the drugs of choice.
3. Can D/C mechanical ventilation when requirement for resting minute ventilation is low (< 10 liters) and when patient can demonstrate reserve by more than doubling the resting value on command.

INTRACTABLE ASTHMA

   Poor communication between physician and patient is probably the primary reason for lack of compliance with asthma therapy. The complicated nature of the drug regimen and the potential side effects of the various medications makes it necessary for the patient to be very knowledgeable about the medication he is taking, the potential side effects and how to adjust his medi-- cations if he does develop significant side effects. Some patients will discontinue all medicines because of increasing frustration due to the restrictions placed on their lives by asthma. Often patients will get into a pattern of repeated Emergency Room visits for acute

treatment of attacks without establishing a relationship with one physician who can serve as a coordinator
of the therapeutic program.

REFERENCES

Saunders, N.A., McFadden, E.R: Asthma-An Update, Dis-
ease-a-Month XXIV: 1-49, Year Book Medical Publish-
ers, Inc., Chicago, 1978.
Farr, R.S: Asthma in Adults: The Ambulatory Patient,
Hospital Practice, April, 1978.
Reed, C.E. and Townley, R.G: Asthma-Classification
and Pathogenesis, in Allergy Principles and Practice,
Middleton, E., Reed, C.E. and Ellis, E.F. (eds),
C.V. Mosby Co., Saint Louis, 1978.
Spector, S.L. and Farr, R.S: The Heterogeneity of
Asthmatic Patients--an Individualized Approach to
Diagnosis and Treatment, J. Allergy Clin. Immunol.
57:499-511, 1976.
Patterson, R., Suszko, I.M. and Harris, K.E: The in
vivo Transfer of Antigen-Induced Airway Reactions
by Bronchial Lumen Cells, J. Clin. Invest. 62:519-
524, 1978.
English, G.M: Nasal Polyps and Sinusitis, in Allergy
Principles and Practice, Middleton, E., Reed, C.E.
and Ellis, E.F. (eds), C.V. Mosby Co., Saint Louis,
1978.
Strauss, R.H. et al: Enhancement of Exercise-Induced
Asthma by Cold Air, N. Eng. J. Med. 297:743-747,
1977.
Strauss, R.H. et al: Influence of Heat and Humidity
on the Airway Obstruction Induced by Exercise in
Asthma, J. Clin. Invest. 61:433-440, 1978.
Jenne, J.W., Wyzer, E., Rood, F.S. and MacDonald,
F.M: Pharmacokinetics of Theophylline, Clin. Phar-
macol. Ther. 13:349-360, 1972.
Bernstein, I.L. et al: Therapy with Cromolyn Sodium,
Ann. Intern. Med. 89:228-233, 1978.
Jusko, W.J. et al: Intravenous Theophylline Therapy:
Nomogram Guidelines, Ann. Intern. Med. 86:400-404,
1977.
Rebuck, A.S. and Read, J: Assessment and Management
of Severe Asthma, Am. J. Med. 51:788-798, 1971.

McFadden, E.R. et al: Acute Bronchial Asthma-- Relations Between Clinical and Physiological Manifestations, N. Eng. J. Med. 288:221-225, 1973.
Wolfe, J.D. et al: Bronchodilator Effects of Terbutaline and Aminophylline Alone and in Combination in Asthmatic Patients, N. Eng. J. Med. 298:363-367, 1978.
Kelsen, S.G. et al: Emergency Room Assessment and Treatment of Patients with Acute Asthma--Adequacy of the Conventional Approach, Am.J.Med. 64:622-628, 1978.
Scoggin, C.H. Sahn, S.A. and Petty, TL: Status Asthmaticus--A Nine Year Experience, JAMA 238:1158-1162, 1977.
Reisman, R.E: Asthma Induced by Adrenergic Aerosols (Abst), J. Allergy 45:108-109, 1970.
Rosenberg, M., Patterson, R., Mintzer, R., Cooper, B.J., Roberts, M. and Harris, K.E: Clinical and Immunologic Criteria for the Diagnosis of Allergic Bronchopulmonary Aspergillosis, Ann. Intern. Med. 86:405-414, 1977.

Joseph M. Young

THEOPHYLLINE IN THE TREATMENT
OF ASTHMA

INTRODUCTION

Although theophylline has been effectively employed
in the treatment of asthma for over forty years, the
vast majority of physicians, until relatively recently,
prescribed it orally only in fixed combination pills
with some   ephedrine and phenobarbital. However, the
last several years have witnessed a marked deviation
from this pattern and a virtual explosion in single entity theophylline preparations. The reasons for these
changes are multiple, but include: 1) a more complete
understanding of the pharmacology and pharmaco-kinetics
of theophylline; 2) the emergence of pure beta agonists,
i.e. metaproteroneol, terbutaline; and 3) disenchant-
ment not only with ephedrine sulphate as a broncodila-
tor, but more importantly, with the entire philosophy
of fixed combination therapy.

Theophylline is a methylated xanthine, a group of
substances which include theobromine and caffeine, and
which share several pharmacologic properties. This
group stimulates both skeletal muscle and the central
nervous system; has an inotropic and chronotropic
effect on cardiac muscle; and relaxes smooth muscle,
especially bronchial musculature. These effects are
produced with varying intensity depending on the tissue studied. Caffeine, for example, is primarily a
central nervous system and skeletal muscle stimulant,
while theophylline is most potent 'on smooth and cardiac
muscle. Theobromine, in contrast, has less intensive
effects in all areas.

THERAPEUTIC OBSERVATIONS

The therapeutic efficacy of theophylline is best

understood on a cellular level. Current formulation
identifies cyclic AMP as the critical component which
modulates multiple cell functions. Although production
of cyclic AMP is usually associated with secretory processes, the high levels produced in inflammation inhibit
the release of mediators of the inflammatory response.
Theophylline is a potent inhibitor of cyclic nucleotide
phosphodiesterases, a family of enzymes responsible for
the conversion of cyclic AMP to 5' AMP, thereby eleva-
ting intracellular levels. Beta agonists also elevate
cyclic AMP but function at another metabolic step and,
for this reason, their clinical effects are either add-
itive or synergistic.
     The structural formula of hydrous 1-3 dimethylxan-
thine i.e. theophylline, is shown in Figure 1.

$$H_3C-N-C=O$$
$$O=C \quad C-NH$$
$$H_3C-N-C-N{\nearrow}^{CH} \cdot H_2O$$

Theophylline

Initial pharmacologic studies indicated that the drug
was erratically absorbed. This was attributed to poor
solubility characteristics and led to the use of theophylline salts, the commonest of which is aminophylline
(theophylline ethylenediamine). More recent studies
have indicated that gastrointestinal absorption is relatively uniform using anhydrous preparations or salts.
Moreover, the critical determinant of serum levels is
the quantity of anhydrous theophylline presented to the
gastrointestinal tract. In fact, pharmaceutical pro-

cesses that enhance tablet disintegration may be the
more important variable in currently marketed preparations. Peak plasma levels occur at 30-60 minutes after
liquid preparations and at approximately 60-90 minutes
when given in solid form. The presence of food seems
of little consequence. Table 1 lists the major theophylline salts and the percentage of anhydrous theophylline they contain. This is extremely important
since the amount prescribed relates to the salt and not
free theophylline. For example, a patient controlled on
theophylline which is pure anhydrous theophylline, 200
mgs every six hours, if switched to "Choledyl", (theophylline oxytriphylline 200),will only be receiving 128
mgs of anhydrous theophylline per dose. Thus for equi-
valency and effectiveness, a patient should receive
Choledyl 400 mgs, three times per day or Choledyl 200
mgs every three to four hours or six times per day.

TABLE 1

Preparation	% Free Theophylline
Anhydrous theophylline	100
Theophylline H_2O	91
Aminophylline	79
Theophylline ethanolamine	75
Dyphylline	72
Ambuphylline	67
Oxtriphylline	64
Theophylline sodium salicylate	47

The finding that improvement in pulmonary function
correlates directly with plasma theophylline levels
combined with readily available methods to measure plasma theophylline has led to extensive literature on this
topic. Determination of critical plasma levels, distribution, and rates of metabolism and excretion in
various subpopulations have created a finely tuned allo-
rhythm for administration. Intravenous or orally administered theophylline peaks in the central (plasma)
compartment and declines as it is distributed to the
peripheral (tissue) compartment. The distribution is
rapid and, for this reason, theophylline behaves like a
one compartment drug. This allows for calculation of
loading and maintenance doses. Ideal plasma theophyl-

line levels are between 10-20 µg/ml, with little demonstrable effect on airway function below 10 µg/ml and
toxicity usually, but not inevitably, occurring above
20 µg/ml. Loading and maintenance doses are calculated
to reach peak levels of below 20 µg/ml, but above 10 µg/
ml.

The principal means of elimination of theophylline
is hepatic biotransformation. Renal clearance accounts
for only 10% of an administered dose and, therefore,
little adaptation is required in the presence of renal
failure. Marked individual variability in the metabolic
degradation exists and even this is modulated by various
factors such as age, illness and cigarette smoking.
Children eliminate the drug much more rapidly than
adults, with adolescents falling somewhere in between
(Table 2). On a mg/kg basis, children therefore require
much higher maintenance doses. Liver disease and
cardiac failure result in reduced clearance, while cigarette smoking increases clearance. Although theophylline
is a methylated xanthine, xanthine oxidase is not involved in its degradation; thus allopurinol does not
effect its transformation. Enzyme induction by phenobarbital may increase clearance, but studies utilizing
doses normally taken in fixed combinations have not
shown any significant change in the plasma half-life of
theophylline

TABLE 2
Oral Dosage to Achieve Serum Concentrations of 10µg/ml

	Young children	Older children	Adults
Anhydrous Theophylline (mg/kg/6 hrs)	5.6	4.6	3.1
Aminophylline (mg/kg/6 hrs)	7.0	5.8	3.9

TOXICITY

Theophylline has a low therapeutic index, i.e. a
narrow range between clinically effective and toxic
levels. Generally, toxicity is almost always due to
overdoseage; however in adults, toxicity also seems to
occur in those with underlying liver and cardiac disorders. The physician, however, must distinguish between adverse and toxic effects; these may be qualita-

tively similar, but differ in severity. Normally, oral
theophylline preparations produce some degree of gastric
irritation, occasional abdominal cramping and diarrhea
and, rarely, severe nausea and vomiting. These latter
symptoms may, in fact, be due not to gastrointestinal
effects, but rather direct stimulation of the medulla.
Restlessness, irritability and insomnia are common CNS
symptoms which may be potentiated by the simultaneous
use of either ephedrine or newer beta agonists.
Seizures and hypothermia are signs of severe intoxica-
tion. Theophylline usually elevates the pulse rate,
increases cardiac output and, therefore, increases renal
blood flow, producing diuresis. This may lead to mild
to moderate dehydration which may be significant, particularly in children. Signs of cardiac toxicity
include tachycardia, and rhythm disturbances. In fact,
theophylline, even in non-toxic doses, increases cardiac
irritability and should be used with caution in patients
with underlying arrhythmias.

DOSAGE

     Adult asthmatics are usually begun on an equivalent
of 100-150 mgs of anhydrous theophylline four times a
day. In the absence of significant side effects, the
doseage may be doubled and the dosing interval lengthened, i.e. 200 mgs t.i.d. Routine plasma levels are usually not required to follow these incremental changes.
Minor variations, such as higher early morning dose to
re-establish loading, or a high evening dose for nocturnal asthma is occasionally recommended.
     Liquid preparations are almost always utilized in
young children. Alcohol does not appreciably alter
absorption, but non-ethanolic solutions are preferred
in severe asthmatics who require round the clock therapy.
Dosing intervals are usually shorter, i.e. every three
to four hours, due to earlier peak levels with liquid
preparations and more rapid elimination rates in children. A normogram for calculation of I.V. doseages
based on age and weight is shown in Table 3; however,
plasma levels are more frequently required to achieve
a maximal therapeutic response. Rectal administration
is not generally recommended. Absorption is more predictable when using solutions than with suppositories.

106

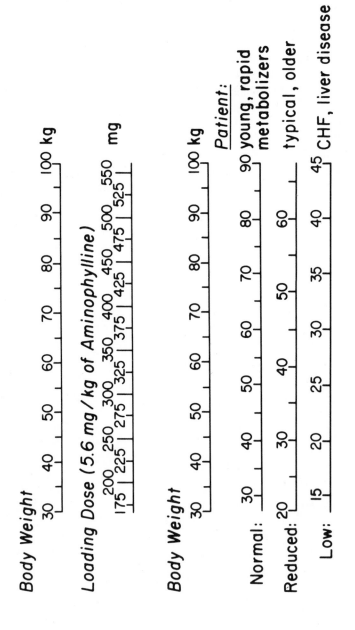

TABLE 3: Theophylline doseage normogram

Chronic use frequently leads to proctitis and rectal
bleeding.

Intravenous administration is generally required in
the severe asthmatic, particularly in status asthmaticus. The doseage schedules printed in this article are
applicable to both oral and intravenous administration.
Theophylline should never be given via a central venous
catheter since this markedly potentiates the cardiac
effects and frequently leads to hypotension. Once a
loading dose is given over a short period of time, then
constant intravenous infusion is preferred to a periodic
bolus. There are no known antidotes for theophylline.
Treatment of the severely toxic patient consists of
fluids to correct dehydration and for their dilutional
effect. Otherwise, measures are supportive although
cardiac rhythm should be monitored until plasma theophylline levels return to normal.

REFERENCES

Goodman, L.S. and Gilman, A., editors: The pharmacolog-
    ical basis of therapeutics. 5th ed. Macmillan, Inc.
    N.Y. 1975.
Ellis, E.F., and Eddy, E.O.: Anhydrous theophylline ˙
    equivalence of commercial theophylline formulations.
    J. Allergy Clin. Immunol. 53: 116, 1974.
Ellis, E.F., Koysooko, R., and Levy, G.: Pharmacokine-
    tics of theophylline in children with asthma.
    Pediatrics. 58: 542, 1976.
Jacobs, M.H., Senior, R.M., and Kessler, G.: Clinical
    experience with theophylline: Relationships between
    dosage, serum concentration and toxicity. J.A.M.A.
    235: 1983, 1976.
Mitenko, P.A. and Ogilvie, R.I.: Pharmacokinetics of
    intravenous theophylline. Clin. Pharmacol. Ther.
    14: 509, 1973.
Piafky, K.M., and Ogilvie, R.I.: Dosage of theophylline
    in bronchial asthma. N. Eng. J. Med. 292: 1218,
    1975.
Jenne, J.W., Wyze, E., Rood, F.S., and MacDonald, F.M.:
    Pharmacokinetics of theophylline: Application to ad-
    justment of the clinical dose of aminophylline. Clin.
    Pharmacol. Ther. 13: 349, 1972.

Martin D. Valentine

IMMUNOTHERAPY OF ALLERGIC
RESPIRATORY DISEASE

INTRODUCTION

Initial attempts at immunization to relieve
symptoms of hay fever were based on the knowledge that
antisera specifically directed against toxic materials
could neutralize such toxins. Indeed it was felt that
pollen grains contained materials which were toxic to
susceptible individuals and that an antitoxin could be
used to neutralize such effects. Thus, patients were
immunized with the intention of having the immunized
individuals develop active immunity; when these patients improved, it was concluded that this theory had
been validated. At about this time, investigators
began to appreciate the significance of the immunizing
process in the development of the state of anaphylactic
susceptibility in laboratory animals. "Anaphylaxis,"
first thought to be the result of lowered resistance
in animals to exogenous toxic material, was found
instead to be the result of heightened sensitivity due
to repeated administration of antigens. An intracutaneous injection of a very small amount of antigen
was found to result in a wheal and erythema in sensitive animals. It was found that the hypersensitive
state could be abrogated by the repeated administration
of antigen doses, each in itself too small to evoke any
signs or symptoms of anaphylaxis. Animals rendered
first hypersensitive and subsequently insensitive were
said to be "desensitized," and this condition was
accompanied by a loss of the previously positive skin
test. Soon after Noon and Freeman reported their
success, Cooke described the successful treatment of
114 patients treated for asthma and hay fever due to
pollen hypersensitivity. Cooke, as well as others,

found that clinical improvement occurred without change
in skin test reactivity, and drew a distinction between
desensitization, such as could be established in an
animal model, and the state in man following injections
of pollen extract. As the term "desensitization" did
not seem applicable to the state induced in man, the
new term, "hyposensitization," was coined to describe
the process of therapeutic allergen administration.

SKIN TESTING

     It was not until the description of the passive
transfer of specific sensitivity in normal human skin
that a means for demonstrating changes in the patient's
allergic state was found. The technique as it was
originally described, and as it may (with few modifications, to insure sterility and to avoid transfer of
hepatitis virus) be performed today, involved first
the identification of an individual, himself non-atopic
(and therefore negative upon direct skin-testing with
appropriate allergens), whose skin could be locally
"sensitized" by the intracutaneous administration of a
fraction of a milliliter of serum obtained from a
person with one or more specific known allergies. The
process of passive sensitization itself appears to
take some time (24 to 72 hours) to accomplish, but
once established, persists for up to six weeks. Proof
of passive sensitization is obtained by intracutaneous
challenge of skin sites so prepared, as well as
challenge of control (unsensitized) sites with the
relevant allergen. The concentration of allergen
required to elicit a positive test at a passively
sensitized site is generally 10 to 50-fold greater than
that required to elicit a positive direct skin test in
the sensitive donor.
     Using this technique, it was thus possible to show
in individuals who had been successfully treated with
pollen extract injections, that a gradual change
occurred in the capacity of their sera to sensitize
non-allergic recipient skin sites. This change consisted in an apparent reduction in sensitizing ability,
particularly evident in the weaker dilutions of donor
serum. The substance which caused passive sensitization was referred to as "reagin," or "reaginic anti-

body." Changes in the titer of reaginic antibody were
often not spectacular, and the passive transfer technique was subsequently used to demonstrate another,
perhaps more dramatic change: the appearance in the
serum of treated individuals of a substance called
"blocking" antibody.

If multiple sites are sensitized in a recipient,
one may determine whether serum from an immunized
individual contains "blocking" antibody. This can be
done by brief incubation of potentially immune serum
with the antigen prior to challenge of passively
sensitized skin sites with the antigen-immune serum
mixture. If the "immune" serum effects an increase
in the minimum concentration of antigen required to
elicit a positive test at a passively sensitized skin
site, then "blocking antibody" actively has been
functionally demonstrated. Immune sera can be
greatly diluted while still retaining blocking activity;
the "titer" of blocking antibody may be expressed as
the reciprocal of the greatest dilution of immune serum
which is capable of diminishing the reaction to antigen at a passively sensitized site.

REAGINIC ANTIBODY

Functional evidence of the existence of reaginic
and blocking antibody were thus found considerably
before electrophoretic and chromatographic techniques
were available to allow the separation and purification
of these immunoglobulin classes (IgE and IgG) from
serum. In the past decade, elucidation of the biochemical events which are involved in acute allergic
reactions has allowed allergists and immunologists to
investigate how immunotherapy, as well as pharmacologic
therapy, may influence the outcome of the allergic
reaction in vitro.

There is a consensus that reaginic antibody--the
heat-labile substance in human serum that can sensitize
recipient primate skin to subsequent antigen challenge—
belongs to the IgE class of immunoglobulins. Rare
reports of IgG with reaginic activity in man have been
heard, although the preponderance of evidence supports
IgE as the major, if not sole, culprit in human immediate hypersensitivity and anaphylaxis. In some sub-

primate mammals, special sub-classes of IgG may possess
mast-cell sensitizing ability. In man, the correlation
between blocking antibody and IgG is so close as to
discourage speculation regarding blocking activity in
other immunoglobulin classes. Nevertheless, it is
tempting to speculate that if blocking activity were
present in IgA secretory antibodies, such activity
would teleologically possess some evolutionary advan-
tages.

Thus, although a number of controlled clinical
studies have been performed in Europe and the United
States in the past 25 years which demonstrate unequivocally that immunization with reasonably well-defined
antigenic material is effective in reducing symptoms
in patients with allergic respiratory disease, there
is considerably less certainty regarding the mechanism
for improvement in symptoms after immunization is
applied. A number of parameters have been considered:
not only the blocking antibody response, which has been
appreciated since the days of Cooke, but also specific
titers of IgE against antigens related to the allergic
condition; sensitivity of the IgE-sensitized cells to
antigen challenge; and speculatively, other as yet
undescribed and therefore unappreciated factors.

It seems clear that no patient immunized with an
antigen such as ragweed or grass pollen extract fails
to respond with an IgG response. However, it has been
appreciated for at least 60 years that the magnitude
of the IgG response, whether measured by specific
radioimmunoassay or functionally by capacity of immune
serum to block antigen-induced skin tests or leukocyte
histamine release does not correlate as well as would
be hoped with the degree of symptomatic relief
experienced by patients. That is to say, it can be
shown that some patients who have little symptomatic
relief from immunization have made extremely high
titers of blocking antibody; and the converse also may
be true. Thus, other explanations for loss of clinical symptoms has been sought, and it can be shown that
after immunotherapy has been conducted for a period of
time the IgE-sensitized cells become less sensitive
to antigen challenge: that is, it requires a larger dose
of antigen to effect the same degree of histamine
release that formerly, in the same patient, was effect-

ed by a relatively small dose of antigen. This is
more easily appreciated in in vitro systems utilizing
blood basophils, possibly because in vitro techniques
have often lent themselves more easily to precise
quantitation than biological techniques involving the
whole organism, such as skin testing. However, the
correlation between decrease in cell sensitivity and
symptom relief is not the whole answer, nor does the
answer reside in the apparent drop in circulating
antigen-specific IgE that occurs after successful
immunotherapy. Some years ago, Levy made an interesting and at that time hopeful discovery in antigen-
immunized children; he was able to find children whose
blood basophils not only became less sensitive, but
became absolutely insensitive to antigen challenge--
they failed to release histamine regardless of the
dose of antigen chosen. In a sense, histamine release
mechanism in the cells of these children appeared to
have been "turned off." Whether such a phenomenon is
antigen-specific or whether it is totally non-specific
has not adequately been explored, since attempts at
repeating this experiment have not met with success
and similar results have not been seen in adults.

CLINICAL OBSERVATIONS

Regardless of the mechanism responsible for improvement of symptoms in immunotherapy, it is quite clear
that when patients whose well-defined seasonal symptoms
of allergic rhinitis are immunized with potent antigens,
they do benefit from specific immunotherapy. Norman
and Lichtenstein, using a meticulously controlled
method involving comparison of placebo-immunized
patients with allergen-treated patients, showed that
a specifically treated group could not be distinguished
from an allergen-immunized group unless a cumulative
antigen dose somewhat larger than had been customary
was used. Nearly as important as this demonstration
of efficacy was the demonstration that significant
numbers of patients in placebo-treated groups felt
improved as a result of their treatment. This under-
lined an observation which can never be too greatly
stressed; that although it is a laudable achievement
if a physician helps his patient feel better, it is

even more laudable if the physician knows whether the
result is placebo-induced or the result of some real
therapeutic intervention with specific consequences.

Considerably more debate has arisen around the
question of whether other respiratory disease, e.g.
asthma, benefits from immunotherapy. A number of
problems have surrounded the role of immunotherapy in
asthma, not the least of which is the inability of
"experts" to define asthma. Some experts regard asthma
not as a single entity but as a final clinical expression which is composed of multiple physiological variables. Regardless of the final definition of asthma,
if one is ever obtained, it does seem clear that some
individuals who have asthma defined as reversible
obstructive airway disease have low serum IgE levels;
have negative skin tests; have non-seasonal histories
with respect to antigen exposure; and otherwise have
no manifestations that one would attribute to antigen
exposure.

It did seem reasonable, however, to attempt to
study "allergic asthma" by enlisting patients who
reported seasonal symptoms during the ragweed season
and who have corroborative positive skin tests to
significantly small concentrations of ragweed antigen.
It was proposed to study such patients by a variety of
techniques, including evaluation of symptoms diaries
in control and treated groups, determination of
sensitivity by inhalation challenge before and after
therapy of both placebo and treated patients, and
measurement of antibody and cellular responses.

Such studies are fraught with many difficulties
and a number of interesting observations have been made
in the course of trying to conduct such studies. These
include the observation that patients with allergic
rhinitis due to ragweed can be shown to have an increase in airway resistance after the inhalation of
allergen solution, suggesting that although they don't
have "asthma" that they certainly do have some sort
of airway response when aerosolized allergen is inhaled.
Furthermore, patients with asthma or with allergic
rhinitis can be given whole pollen grains to inhale
and are found to have grains deposited in the upper
airway but not in the lower airway; none of these
patients will develop airways responses to such

inhalation. In a study conducted by Drs. Bruce and
Norman, it was found that patients who were carefully
selected on the basis of a history of seasonal asthma
and ragweed sensitivity were found to lack the seasonal
peak in symptoms that occurs in ragweed hay fever
patients as they were observed through the course of
several seasons. Such a lack in symptomatology during
the putatively responsible allergen season makes it
very difficult to estimate the efficacy of a mode of
therapy aimed at preventing this peak in symptoms.

Studies have been reported in the past of both a
negative and positive nature with respect to immunotherapy in asthma, and although certain of these
studies appear to be quite well done, they are few and
far between. It is therefore fair to say that at this
point it is much more difficult to reach conclusions
regarding the efficacy of immunotherapy in asthma than
it has been to reach conclusions about this treatment
for allergic rhinoconjunctivitis.

REFERENCES

Aas K: Hyposensitization in house dust allergy asthma.
    Acta Paediatr Scand 60: 264, 1971.
Bruce CA, Norman PS, Rosenthal RR and Lichtenstein LM:
    The role of ragweed pollen in autumnal asthma. J
    Allergy Clin Immunol 59: 449-459, 1977.
Bruce CA, Rosenthal RR, Lichtenstein LM, and Norman PS:
    Diagnostic tests in ragweed allergic asthma: A
    comparison of direct skin tests, leukocyte hista-
    mine release and bronchial challenge. J Allergy
    Clin Immunol 53: 230, 1974.
Bruce CA, Rosenthal RR, Lichtenstein LM and Norman PS:
    Quantitative inhalation bronchial challenge in
    ragweed hay fever patients: A comparison with
    ragweed allergic asthmatics. J Allergy Clin
    Immunol 56: 331-337, 1975.
Cooke RA: Active immunization in hay fever. Laryngo-
    scope 25: 108, 1915.
Cooke RA: Studies in specific hypersensitiveness. IX.
    On the phenomenon of hypersensitization (the
    clinically lessened sensitiveness of allergy). J
    Immunol 7: 219, 1922.

Cooke RA, Barnard JH, Hebald S and Stull A: Serologic
    evidence of immunity with coexisting sensitization
    in a type of human allergy (hay fever). J Exp
    Med 62: 733, 1935.
Freeman J and Noon L: Further observations on the
    treatment of hay fever by hypodermic inoculations
    of pollen vaccine. Lancet 2: 814, 1911.
Johnstone DE: Value of hyposensitization therapy for
    perennial bronchial asthma in children. Pediatrics
    27: 39, 1961.
Noon L: Prophylactic inoculation against hay fever.
    Lancet 1: 1572, 1911.
Norman PS, Winkenwerder W, and Lichtenstein L: Immuno-
    therapy of hay fever with ragweed antigen E:
    Comparisons with whole pollen extract and placebos.
    J Allergy 42: 93, 1968.
Norman PS, Winkenwerder WL, and Lichtenstein LM: Trials
    of alum-precipitated pollen extracts in the treat-
    ment of hay fever. J Allergy Clin Immunol 50:
    31, 1972.
Portier P and Richet C: D L'action anaphylactique de
    certaines venins. Compt Redn Soc Biol 54: 170,
    1902.
Prausnitz C and Küstner J: Studien Über die ueberemp-
    findlichkeit. Cent Backt 86: 160, 1921.
Sadan N, Rhyne MB, Mellits D, et al: Immunotherapy of
    pollinosis in children: An investigation of the
    immunologic basis of clinical improvement. N
    Engl J Med 280: 623, 1969.
Sherman WB: Changes in serologic reactions and tissue
    sensitivity in hay fever patients during the early
    months of treatment. J Immunol 40: 289, 1941.
Sherman WB: Reaginic and blocking antibodies. J
    Allergy 28: 62, 1957.

Harold S. Novey

SELECTED ALLERGIC DISEASES OF THE LUNG:
HYPERSENSITIVITY PNEUMONITIS, ALLERGIC BRONCHOPULMONARY
ASPERGILLOSIS, OCCUPATIONAL ASTHMA

INTRODUCTION

The lung is subject to a number of pathological
changes influenced to a larger or smaller degree by immunological reactivity. The respiratory tract is a
principal contact between man's internal and external
environment by virtue of the inspiration and expiration
of some 10,000 liters of ambient air every day. In the
process of absorbing oxygen and releasing carbon dioxide, the respiratory system must cope with the almost
limitless, additional substances in that air, other
gases, liquids, and particles. The lung is comparable
to the lymphoid organs as a source of immuno-competent
cells and immune mediators, and thus it is fertile
ground for immunoactivity. Predominantly, this arena
for interaction between foreign matter with antigenic
qualities and local antibodies and immunocytes including T lymphocytes and macrophages promotes clinical immunity, but for various and often unexplained reasons,
clinical hypersensitivity syndromes also occur.
The three conditions to be considered here, namely:
hypersensitivity pneumonitis (HP), allergic bronchopulmonary aspergillosis (APBA), and occupational asthma
(OA) have in common immunoreactivity to inhalant antigens. The inhalants may be natural or synthetic, are
mainly particulates, and probably in the size range of
0.5 - 3.0 u in diameter.
In occupational asthma, the bronchi are mainly affected, while in HP and APBA there is often damage not
only to the airways but also to pulmonary interstitium
and alveoli.

HYPERSENSITIVITY PNEUMONITIS

This term encompasses a group of pulmonary interstitial inflammatory diseases associated with sensitization to inhaled organic dusts. It has been used inter-
changeably with extrinsic allergic alveolitis, a term
proposed by Pepys in 1969. Although these names are
relatively new, recognition of the clinical entities
and even their relationship to allergic reactions are
not. Thus, Farmer's lung was reported in 1958, Mushroom worker's lung in 1959, and Pigeon breeder's lung
in 1965. A growing list of related diseases were subsequently reported and these have been classified together as hypersensitivity pneumonitides. (Table 1)
They share common clinical, immunological and histolo-
gical features but none of these findings are unique
or pathognomic, and thus this grouping, while helpful
as a clinical tool, awaits more precise definition.

CLINICAL FEATURES

The syndromes manifest in two forms, acute and insidious. There is suggestion that a more intense but
sporadic exposure provokes the acute reaction while
lighter but continuous exposures are responsible for
the insidious form. As examples, the pigeon fancier
who irregularly enters his coop containing 50 birds
will more often present with acute symptoms, while the
person with a single parakeet or budgerigar at home
will more likely develop the insidious type. The acute
form begins some four to nine hours after the exposure
and presents as a classical bacterial like pneumonia
with fever, chills, malaise, cough, dyspnea, and chest
pain. Physical examination uncovers fever from 101°
to 103°, localized râles, tachycardia and tachypnea.
A complete blood count will show a mild to moderate
leucocytosis with a shift to the left but without consistent eosinophilia. Cultures of secretions will not
yield pathogenic organisms. The x-ray findings of the
lungs may be normal but more often show fine to coarse
nodular densities compatible with interstial or alveolar involvement without areas of predilection.
Typically the entire episode will remit within 24 hours
or less, only to recur on subsequent exposure.

TABLE 1
Etiologic Agents in Hypersensitivity Pneumonitis

Disease	Exposure	Antigen
Farmer's lung	Moldy hay and corn	Thermophilic actinomycetes
Mushroom worker's lung	Compost	Micropolyspora faeni
Bagassosis	Moldy bagasse (sugar cane residue)	Thermoactinomyces vulgaris
Humidifier or Air Conditioner lung	Contaminated forced air system	Thermoactinomyces saccharii
Bird handler's lung	Pigeons, parakeets, chickens, turkeys, cockatiels, parrots	Avian proteins
Detergent worker's lung	Laundry detergent manufacture	Bacillus subtilis enzymes
Maple bark stripper's lung	Moldy bark	Cryptostroma corticale
Malt worker's lung	Moldy barley and hops	Aspergillus clavatus
Sequoiosis	Moldy redwood dust	Aureobasidium pulliulans
Paprika splitter's lung	Paprika dust	Mucor stolonifer
Wheat weevil disease	Wheat flour weevils	Sitophilus granarius
Cheese worker's lung	Cheese mold	Penicillium caseii
Suberosis	Moldy cork	Penicillium sp.
Pituitary snuff lung	Porcine, bovine pituitary	Porcine, bovine proteins

The insidious form presents as a step wise incre-
ment in symptoms. The patient is aware of a gradual
decrease in tolerance to physical activity. Initially,
he notices more dyspnea during a sports activity, for
example, later dyspnea on running, then walking uphill,
and finally from routine physical exertion. During
this period, which may extend over several months, he
develops a dry cough, that progresses to a daily cough
productive of clear, mucoid sputum. Weight loss without evident anorexia occurs. Physical examination of
the patient may be normal at this stage. X-ray findings will depend on the degree of interstitial involvement and may not be considered abnormal until significant pulmonary fibrosis has resulted. Pulmonary function tests are often more helpful in confirming pulmonary pathology, especially when tests for arterial blood
gases and diffusing capacity are performed. While during an acute reaction spirometric and lung volume
measurements usually reveal restrictive defects in the
form of decreased vital capacity and compliance, the
insidious type may show only hypoxemia or decreased
diffusion capacity during the earlier stages.

HISTOPATHOLOGIC FEATURES

A few lung biopsy specimens have been obtained
shortly after the acute onset of symptoms in farmers
exposed to inhalants from moldy hay. These showed intensive infiltration of granulocytes, monocytes, and
plasma cells around small to medium blood vessels and
alveoli. Alveolar walls appeared thickened, capillaries congested, but there were no thrombi or tissue ne-
crosis. Most examinations of specimens in the chronic
stage report interstitial pneumonitis with infiltrates
predominantly of lymphocytes in alveolar walls, and
interstitial fibrosis with granuloma formation but no
signs of the vasculitis found in the acute type.
Whether the latter represents progression from an acute
stage is not established.

IMMUNOPATHOGENIC FEATURES

The following findings suggest an immunological
basis for this group of diseases: exacerbations as-

sociated with both natural exposures and laboratory
bronchial challenges, elevated IgG and IgM levels, deposition of IgG, M,A, and complement components in
lung sections that show vasculitis, elution of specific
antigen from these deposits in a few cases, presence of
precipitating antibodies to extracts of the provoking
agents (circulating immune complexes have not been reported as yet), that tend to disappear on removal from
exposure and disease remission. Animal models include
a naturally occurring disease in cows, and the relative ease of producing pulmonary lesions with inhalation or injection techniques using either bovine serum
albumin or extracts of the agents associated with human HP in various species from mice to monkeys. Although there is predominant evidence of an immune complex, Type III mechanism, findings in the various animal models have prompted investigators to evoke Type
I, II, and IV immunopathogenic mechanisms.

DIFFERENTIAL DIAGNOSIS

This will include any of the acute or chronic interstitial pulmonary diseases in Table 2 . The diagnosis
is less difficult to suspect in the acute form associated with an occupational or avocational exposure
such as the farmer pitching hay after a rain, or the
pigeon breeder cleaning his coop. It is when association with a specific exposure is not present that the
diagnosis presents a major problem. In that case, it
may involve exclusion of other diseases, a search for
fungal contamination in the home or office environment,
and a serological screening for precipitins to some of
the antigens listed in Table 1.

DIAGNOSIS

The typical histories, a high index of suspicion,
the absence of infectious agents, radiological and pulmonary function abnormalities will point the way to
the diagnosis. The presence of serum precipitins to
antigens in the environment is a helpful confirmatory
finding. More conclusive is the absence of recurring
attacks or improvement of the insidious form upon removal from exposures, together with disappearance of

TABLE 2
Hypersensitivity Pneumonitis: Differential Diagnosis

Acute Onset	Insidious Onset
Asthma	Chronic obstructive lung disease
Infectious processes	Effects of noxious agents
Bronchopneumonia	Beryllium
Influenza	Asbestos
Other viral pneumonias	Diatomaceous earth
Varicella	Talc
Miliary tuberculosis	Silica
Miliary fungous infection	Generalized disease of unknown etiology
Effects of noxious agents	Sarcoidosis
Irritating gases such as chlorine, phosgene, sulfur dioxide, and oxides of nitrogen(silo-filler's disease)	Rheumatoid arthritis, polymyositis, disseminated lupus erythematosus, scleroderma, etc.
Beryllium	Necrotizing granulomatosis
Cotton dust (byssinosis)	Pulmonary histiocytosis
	Lymphogenous carcinomatosis including lymphomas and pulmonary adenomatosis
Bordeaux mixture	Pulmonary alveolar microlithiasis
Epoxy resins	Primary pulmonary hemosiderosis
Generalized systemic disease	Hamman-Rich syndrome
Uremia	Desquamative interstitial pneumonitis
Acute disseminated lupus erythematosus	Chronic eosinophilic pneumonia
Acute polyarteritis nodosa	Radiation pneumonitis
Acute diffuse interstitial fibrosis (Hamman-Rich syndrome)	

the specific serum precipitins. In those relatively
few cases when the diagnosis must be further confirmed
because of problems involving compensation or job and
hobby changes, resort to the risky inhalation challenge
can be made. A lung biopsy may confirm the interstitial inflammatory nature of the disease but not the
etiology. Thus, the diagnosis is made on the basis of
a number of historical, functional, and laboratory
data, none of which are specific in themselves, but
together suggest a definite clinical entity.

TREATMENT

     Milder acute reactions will subside without any
other than supportive measures such as bed rest, oxygen
for hypoxemia, and occasionally broncho-dilators for
any obstructive airway component. In more severe or
persistent cases, hospitalization and the use of steroids are needed. Prednisone in a dosage of about 0.5
mg/kg daily for one to four weeks is usually successful
in hastening recovery of symptoms as well as x-ray and
pulmonary function abnormalities. Of course, the most
effective treatment is prophylactic. The antigen
sources must be identified and preferably completely
removed. Often this is a harder task than it appears.
For the occasional worker or the person with a pet
bird or two, separation from the offender can be easily
affected. However, the breeder of pigeons, or the
racing pigeon enthusiast is loathe to surrender his
hobby. Farmers, ranchers, dairymen, poultry men and
agricultural inspectors are in conflict over risk to
health and risk to livelihood. In such cases, protective measures including filters, air cleaning, changes
in operation need to be instituted on an individual
basis.
     Recognition of this category of diseases has a
special importance in that it identifies cases that
were once labeled idiopathic, diffuse interstitial fibrosis, and its prompt treatment can prevent disabling
pulmonary disease, cor pulmonale, and death.

ALLERGIC BRONCHOPULMONARY ASPERGILLOSIS

This is an inflammatory bronchial and interstitial
lung disease characterized by tissue and blood eosinophilia and associated with immunological responses to
bronchial colonization by members of the fungus genus
Aspergillus. With few exceptions, it occurs in patients with pre-existing asthma. It represents a complication of asthma and is manifest as either an acute
bronchitis or pneumonitis, or in a more chronic form
as a proximal type bronchiectasis, and more rarely as
bronchocentric granulomatosis. Although the syndrome
was first described by Hinson, Moon, and Plummer in
1952, it is probably not a new entity. For many years,
bronchiectasis and transient pulmonary infiltrates with
eosinophilia have been assoicated with asthma. What
is newly recognized is the relationship of these complications with each other and with immunoreactivity to
Aspergillus antigens.

CLINICAL FEATURES

In concert with HP, this syndrome presents a group
of findings, none of which are probably unique, but
in combination do suggest a separate disease. Typically, the patient has had mild to moderate asthma, and
is in the age range of 15-35 years. There is a worsening of his asthma by a bronchitis-like episode, or, less
less often, with pneumonia. He expectorates more vis-
cous and colored sputum than usual, which may contain
1-4 mm. sized golden brown plugs. Initial chest films
often show some degree of consolidation or atelectasis.
In one study of 50 ABPA patients at the Brompton Hospital in England, most had signs of either homogenous
consolidation without shrinkage or bandlike infiltrates.
The larger opacities occurred about equally throughout
the lung zones while the bandlike shadows, likened to
toothpaste, were mostly in the upper lobes. The right
side was more often affected. Serial films confirmed
the transitory and changing nature of the infiltrates,
and in 21% of the abnormal readings, the patient appeared to be asymptomatic. Other descriptions of the
X-ray findings include patchy clouding, nodular, tram-
line, tubular, gloved-finger, and ring shadows. There
was a mean of 5.3 episodes of transient shadows in this

group, but nearly all appeared to have developed permanent X-ray changes. Most of these findings are the
result of dilated proximal bronchi, and, indeed, when
bronchograms are performed in the more chronic cases a
characteristic proximal saccular bronchiectasis is
found. The distal bronchi have a normal calibre. Thus,
there is evidence of recurrence and chronicity of this
disease but the incidence varies greatly among studies,
partly because of differences in populations and diagnostic criteria. Pulmonary function tests will reflect
the degree of asthma and amount of lung tissue damaged,
so there may be combinations of obstructive and restrictive lung changes.

Sputum and peripheral eosinophilia is an invariable
concomitant if the patient is not on steroid medication.
The total eosinophil count is usually over 750 cells,
or over 10% of the leucocyte count, which is not itself
especially elevated. The sedimentation rate by the
Westergren method is nearly always over 20 mm/hour.
The hemoglobulin and hematocrit valves are unaffected.

If the small mucus plugs are obtained, then hyphae
can be identified by staining, and Aspergillus organisms will appear on fungal culture media, such as Sa-
bouraud's or Czapek's agar. But even with repeated
attempts at sputum culture, the yield of positive Aspergillus cultures are no more than 60%. It is felt that
the fungal colonies in the bronchi are distal to the
expectorated sputum in inspissated mucus plugs.

HISTOPATHOLOGIC FEATURES

As may be inferred from the radiographic studies,
pathologic findings may be related either to changes
in the conducting airways or the alveoli, or to both.
Affected bronchi are dilated and filled with inspissated mucus and exudate in which non-invasive fungal hyphae
may be found. The mucosa undergoes squamous metaplasia,
and there is infiltration of eosinophils, lymphocytes,
and plasma cells into the mural portion. The lumina of
alveoli may contain these cells along with large mono-
nuclear cells as in eosinophilic pneumonia. Granulation
tissue protrudes into bronchioles to produce bronchiolitis obliterans. ABPA has been called a condition of

"microimpaction" by Liebow and associates.

In a few patients, after lung biopsy or surgical resection of a lobe, a more virulent expression of the disease has been discovered. A severe necrotizing granulomatous inflammation without vasculitis has occurred called broncho-centric granulomatosis. This condition has been diagnosed also in patients without asthma or ABPA.

IMMUNOPATHOGENIC FEATURES

A number of *in vivo* and *in vitro* immunologic findings are associated with this syndrome.

In vivo: A wheal and flare immediate reaction to a scratch or prick skin test from a 1:50 W/V solution of Aspergillus fumigatus extracts is common. In some, after this initial reaction fades, a second inflammatory one with heat and edema occurs some 4-9 hours later. This Arthus-like response can be more regularly reproduced when the extract at a 1:1000 dilution is applied intracutaneously in the dose of 0.1 ml. Since such a dose could produce an uncomfortably large immediate reaction, pretreatment with an antihistamine may be necessary. The immediate but not the late reaction will then be ablated, while the opposite effect will occur under steroid treatment.

In vitro: Concomitants of the *in vivo* reactions occur in the form of serum IgE antibodies to Aspergillus antigens by a radioallergosorbent test (RAST) and serum precipitins mostly of IgG to Aspergillus antigens by immuno-diffusion tests. The RAST can be obtained commercially, and kits are available for office testing for the precipitins. Several medical centers are actively engaged in performing these tests in their laboratories. As with many allergy extracts, there is no standard Aspergillus antigen so that skin and serological test results will vary with the potency of the material used. Extracts from cultures of any strain of Aspergillus fumigatus will suffice in nearly all cases, but there are occasional exceptions in which the patient will react only to his own strain or species of Aspergillus. Because of this possibility, it would be wise to save positive cultures as a source of new extract testing.

In addition to the finding of specific antibodies
by skin and serological tests, another immunological
component is the presence of high serum levels of IgE.
Although the patient population involved in ABPA tend
to have elevated levels because of the underlying allergic asthma, it appears that the Aspergillus antigens
evoke both specific and non-specific immunoglobulin
responses. The IgE levels are often over 1000 I.U.
while 300 I.U. are the upper levels in unaffected persons.

Evidence that these immunologic abnormalities in
concert may be pathogenic come from studies in which
passively transferred human serum containing both specific IgE antibodies and precipitins but not IgE antibodies alone have resulted in the clinical and histo-
logical picture of ABPA when monkeys so sensitized
were challenged with aerosols of Aspergillus extracts.
Further evidence in humans is the finding of deposits
of IgG, complement, and Aspergillus antigen in the
sites of involvement in resected lung, and of immune
complexes and complement in the circulation. The pre-
vailing opinion is that the pulmonary pathology results
from a combined Type I and Type III reaction to Aspergillus antigen components present in the bronchial
walls and vasculature.

Consideration of the organism will be made here.
The Aspergilli are ubiquitous fungi containing some
160 species with *fumigatus* chiefly responsible for disease in man and animals. It is considered second only
to *Histoplasma capsulatum, Coccidioides immitis,* and
Blastomyces dermatitides as a cause of systemic disease in humans, and it ranks as a major pathogen in
animals, especially birds. Plant sources include compost, hay, straw, decaying leaves and general vegeta-
tive decay, especially when moist. The spores, about
2.5 μ in diameter, are of a suitable size to be deposited in airways. Whether the viscid mucus of asthma
favors their germination and colonization is problema-
tical.

DIFFERENTIAL DIAGNOSIS

Most cases of asthma and eosinophilia will not be
ABPA since these two conditions are so often paired.

Asthma may be complicated by bacterial and viral pneumonias, atelectasis, mucoid impactions and classic bronchiectasis with distal bronchiole involvement. An as-
pergilloma represents colonization in a previously damaged area of the lung. Precipitin activity is pronounced. The finding of a crescent moon translucency
alongside the density (Monod's sign) is almost pathognomonic. Hemoptysis when it occurs is usually more
threatening than in ABPA. Eosinophilic pneumonia has a
characteristic X-ray picture with densities favoring
peripheral and pleural areas and is without the immunological abnormalities of ABPA. Various pulmonary vas-
culitides and granulomatoses such as periarteritis and
Wegener's granulomatosis may confuse but these can often
be differentiated by their extrapulmonary manifestations.
Finally, the hypersensitivity pneumonitides must be considered in the differential diagnosis, see Table 3.

TABLE 3
Characteristics of Allergic Bronchopulmonary Aspergillosis vs. Extrinsic Allergic Alveolitis

	Allergic Bronchopulmonary Aspergillosis	Extrinsic Allergic Alveolitis (hypersensitivity pneumonitis)
Basic Nature	Atopic	Nonatopic
Physical examination	Wheezing	±
Skin test	Dual positivity	±*
X-ray examination	Pulmonary infiltrate --lobar	Pulmonary infiltrates --interstitial
Complications	Atelectasis, bronchiectasis,pulmonary fibrosis (late)	Pulmonary fibrosis
Blood	Eosinophilia	Normal
Sputum	Eosinophilia, mycelia	Normal
Pulmonary function	Obstructive (restrictive, late)	Restrictive
Antibody	Precipitating (IgG) nonprecipitating (IgE)	Precipitating (IgG)
IgE	Elevated	Normal
Proposed immunologic basis	Immediate hypersensitivity and immune complexes	Immune complexes and DH

* Positive reaction is immediate and late in some cases
  of pigeon breeder's lung.

DIAGNOSIS

It should be suspected in patients with asthma,
pulmonary infiltrates, and sputum and blood eosinophilia
or with asthma and recurring bronchitis, or bronchiectasis, or with the expectoration of tiny yellow-brown
mucus plugs.
An initial diagnostic work-up should include:
1. History, physical, environmental survey for
   sources of Aspergillus contamination such as
   mold growth at home or work, humidifiers and
   vaporizers, silage, mulch or compost, live-
   stock, poultry, pet birds, and moldy marihuana
   cigarettes.
2. Chest films; bronchography if evidence of bronchiectasis.
3. CBC, total blood eosinophils, quantitative immunoglobulins (Ig), especially IgE.
4. Sputum culture for Aspergillus and smear for
   eosinophils. Save positive cultures for possible extract preparation.
5. Skin tests. Aspergillus mix, prick with 1:50
   W/V. Check for immediate and delayed reactions.
   If negative for either, retest with 0.1 ml of
   1:1000 intracutaneously.
6. Immunoserological tests. RAST and immunodiffusion tests for specific IgE and precipitating
   antibodies.
Follow-up procedures:
1. Chest films if previously abnormal and during
   exacerbations.
2. Monthly to bimonthly until stable: Total blood
   and sputum eosinophils, sputum cultures for
   fungi, and total IgE and precipitin tests.
The latter two immunological tests appear to predict exacerbations and remissions.

TREATMENT

The natural course of this syndrome is not well established, but there is increasing evidence that a

chronic, sometimes progressive one is not uncommon. If
the first episode is recognized and promptly treated,
and if a known exposure is discovered and eliminated,
the prognosis is most favorable. Treatment includes
bronchodilators, encouragement of expectoration by hydration, chest tapping, and postural drainage. In
some cases, this conservative management has sufficed
to produce remission. It has been shown that steroid
therapy promotes the clearing of the radiographic infiltrates. Whether its effect is due to direct anti-
inflammatory action on the bronchial mucosa, inhibition of immune complex reactivity, or to other modalities is unknown. The dose and duration of steroid
therapy has also not been established. If evidence of
chronicity by history, X-ray, pulmonary function tests,
and culture activity is present, then long-term relatively high-dose steroid therapy has been recommended.
Usually systemic steroids are required, since exacerbations have been reported when patients were switched
to the inhaled forms. Additional measures have been
directed at alleviating the antigenic load by the use
of antifungal agents including amphotericin B, especially
by inhalation, nystatin, clotrimazole, and diiodohydro-
xyquinolone. The results are mostly inconclusive. As
with the steroids, these agents have not been subjected
to good control studies in the treatment of ABPA.
     Although treatment is predominantly medical, sur-
gical intervention has been resorted to in a few cases
of unresolved consolidation of a portion of the lung.
Removal of a severely bronchiectatic or granulomatous
lobe has been of at least temporary benefit.

OCCUPATIONAL ASTHMA

INTRODUCTION

     Occupational asthma refers to those individuals who
develop asthma primarily from exposures at their work
or hobby sites. The term should also include those in-
advertently affected by living in the vicinity or by
contact with the worker. Although occupational asthma
dates at least to Ramazzini's reports in 1700 of asthma
provoked by flour dust in bakers and wig makers, the

sources of exposures seem to be on the increase in recent years. The provoking agents may be divided into
those of <u>animal origin</u> and encompass poultry farmers,
veterinarians, horse, cattle, and sheep breeders, chicken inspectors, laboratory technicians, entomologists,
furriers, and apiarists; <u>vegetable origin</u>: farmers,
hemp workers, grain workers, gardeners, florists, bakers, millers, wood workers; <u>chemicals, inorganic</u>: chro-
mium, platinum, aluminum and nickel factory workers,
electricians, welders, solderers, and <u>chemical, organic</u>:
plastic makers and painters who handle isocyanates,
meat wrappers exposed to polyvinyl fumes, workers in
pharmaceutical plants, tire factory workers, and
workers using enzymes such as trypsin, B. subtilis enzymes and papain. The lists of occupations and agents
are almost endless.

CLINICAL FEATURES

     Occupational asthma does not essentially differ
from any other type of asthma. There are symptoms and
signs of wheezing, dyspnea, chest tightness, cough, tachypnea, and tachycardia. Laboratory tests will reflect
the degree of dehydration with hemoconcentration, the
presence and type of secondary infection with either
leukocytosis or relative leukopenia, and the extent of
eosinophils mobilized in the circulation. Chest films
may show only hyperinflation during the acute, uncom-
plicated attack. Pulmonary function tests will express
the degree of airways narrowing. However, there are
some exceptions to this usual picture.
     Patterns of reactivity: At least three different
non-immediate reactions have been noted after laboratory
challenge to several unrelated occupational agents,
such as bird serum, toluene diisocyanate, flour, papain,
and metallic salts. These controlled observations have
also been encountered in natural clinical settings.
     The first type begins about one hour after exposure
and resolves in about five hours. The second begins
some five hours post exposure, reaches its maximal intensity in the next few fours, and resolves within 24
hours. This is considered the commonest type of reaction by Pepys. The third type begins the evening of the
exposure, often awakens the patient from sleep, and may

recur for several more nights without much daytime distress. The immediate attack is blocked by pretreatment
with bronchodilators and cromlyn sodium, but the non-
immediate attacks are incompletely affected by these
agents and respond best to glucocorticosteroids.

Some subjects will demonstrate combinations of an
immediate and one of the later reactions, called a dual
reaction. The reasons for these patterns are unclear
at present.

Pulmonary function tests: While most acute asthma
represents a combination of large and small airways obstruction with a predominance of the former as measured
by FEV_1, Raw, and PEFR, occupational asthma often ex-
presses in the opposite manner with more profound
changes in measurements such as FEF_{25-75}, closing volumes, and volumes of isoflow with oxygen and helium.

Associated findings: Asthma may not be the sole
clinical expression of the exposure. In the immediate
reactions, asthma may be accompanied by rhinitis, con-
junctivitis, and dermatitis. In the non-immediate
types, systemic complaints have been reported including
myalgia, arthralgia, malaise, and fever. These extra-
bronchial symptoms have occurred from unrelated classes
of agents, i.e., animal, chemical, and plant sources.

HISTOPATHOLOGICAL FEATURES

In contradistinction to patients diagnosed as HP or
ABPA, those suspected of occupational asthma have rarely
been subjected to lung biopsy. Such an invasive procedure would not be expected in a respiratory disease
without radiological signs of a lesion, or when reversibility of symptoms is likely. In the occasional patient
who died, often of some other cause, autopsy findings
consistent with a "chronic asthma" or "chronic bronchitis" were reported. So far as can be determined, no
distinctive pathological changes have been reported in
this category of occupational lung disease, as has, for
example, in coal miners with pneumoconiosis and sili-
cosis.

IMMUNOPATHOGENIC FEATURES

Asthma may occur not only in those who are predis-

posed because they are atopic, but also in apparently
normal persons without a personal or family history of
allergies, or pre-existing IgE antibodies. There is
some evidence that the atopic persons have a more rapid
onset of symptoms following exposures and tend to leave
their jobs sooner. One of the reasons for allergic
type I reactions occurring in non-atopics may be the
nature of the antigen. Castor bean extract used in
fertilizer and animal feeds and present as a contam-
inant in coffee bean sacks is an extremely potent allergen. Intradermal testing with this material has
produced anaphylaxis and death. Asthma in endemic pro-
portions has occurred in the vicinity of castor bean
fertilizer factories even in persons without a prior
history of asthma. As another example, in one study in
which a group of 500 bakers was observed over a six-year
period, 212 developed clear-cut asthma, presumably from
flour dust.

Besides the factor of antigenicity is the status of
the workers' lungs. A prior history of cigarette smoking or frequent respiratory infections or an immunological deficiency may predispose to occupational asthma.

The mechanism of the immediate asthma is considered
to be IgE mediated, and the findings of positive skin,
RAST and PK tests in those afflicted serve as confirmatory evidence. Attempts to passively transfer the
disease with human serum to higher primates have been
successful in a few cases. The mechanism of the non-
immediate attacks of asthma are less clear. There is
evidence that IgE-mediated reactions can be prolonged,
especially when neutrophil chemotactic factors and secondary mediators of inflammation are evoked. The systemic symptoms, the presence of precipitating and other
non-IgE antibodies, and the response to steroids rather
than beta adrenergic agonists have suggested immune
complex and cellular immune mechanisms to others.

Not all the substances responsible for occupational
asthma have antigenic properties. Two other properties
of some agents are considered asthmagenic: 1) irritative, probably acting via vagal receptors in the bronch-
mucosa, and 2) mediator releasing, by the non-immunological disruption of mast cell and basophil granules
that liberate histamine and other vasoactive and inflammatory substances. Examples of the former are fumes

from polyvinyl-chlorides (PVC) when plastic sheets or
labels are heated or from polymerizing catalysts such
as toluene diisocyanate (TDI) used in the manufacture
of polyurethane foam. A portion of the vegetable fiber
called bract in cotton, flax, and soft hemp can release
histamine and is probably at least partly responsible
for the chronic respiratory symptoms of byssinosis. In
Table 4 can be found a list of some of the precipitating
factors and their associate industry in causes of occupational asthma.

DIFFERENTIAL DIAGNOSIS

    This would include all the causes of wheezing dysp-
nea and in any age group since asthma has occurred in
infants and children living near castor bean mills and
poultry farms. Even if asthma has been diagnosed as
caused by pollen and house dust allergens, or the patient has chronic bronchitis or emphysema, some portion
of his bronchospastic disease could be caused or aggra-
vated by the occupational exposure. Thus, the presence
of other causes for asthma does not preclude an occupational component.

DIAGNOSIS

    This depends on a careful, in-depth occupational
and avocational history, knowledge of the various patterns of asthma previously described, and historical
relation between the two. When asthma is worse at work
and improved on vacations, evenings and weekends away
from work, the diagnosis is straightforward. In cases
of nocturnal asthma, one looks for signs of improvement
during vacations and long holiday periods. Other helpful information involves the nature of the industry,
whether it has a known high incidence of asthma, whether
many co-workers are similarly afflicted, and whether
protective measures already installed are being properly used by the worker.
    Physical examination, spirometric tests and response
to bronchodilators serve to confirm the diagnosis of
asthma. Separation from the suspected occupational ha-
zards may be required to confirm that the asthma was
occupational in origin. Unfortunately, in those with

relatively long-standing asthma or with small airway
changes, relief may not be complete after separation.

In such cases in which a diagnosis must be made for
reasons of insurance compensation or the prospect of a
major disruption in a career or livelihood, or when a
new agent is suspected, then challenge and immunological
studies must be undertaken as mentioned for the hypersensitivity pneumonitis group. Such studies are usually
performed at specialized centers for the study of allergic, pulmonary, or occupational diseases. The patient
must be willing to cooperate in studies designed to
provoke his disease and thus have an inherent risk. His
employers must cooperate oftentimes by providing access
to the work site, samples of suspected materials, and
for follow-up evaluation of protective measures.

TREATMENT

Every attempt must be made to alleviate the patient's exposures while at the same time providing symptomatic therapy with bronchodilators, cromlyn sodium,
or, if necessary, inhaled or systemic steroids.

In some cases the patient need not leave his work
permanently if sufficient air cleaning devices, closed
milling and manufacture procedures, substitution of
non-allergic or non-irritative agents, or other such
preventative or protective measures can be effected.
Usually, at least a temporary separation from the work
site is needed until the asthma is brought under control, preferably with a minimum of medication. If, with
the cooperation of occupational health agencies, it can
be shown that the responsible material is no longer present in the worker's ambient air, then he may safely
return to work. In cases where the material is still
present although in lesser amounts, the risk for the
previously symptomatic worker may be high, and return
to work decisions must be considered on an individual
basis. Whether monitoring of immunoserological changes
may be helpful in prognosis as shown for ABPA has not
been clearly established for OA but is being investigated.

SUMMARY

Hypersensitivity pneumonitis, allergic bronchopulmonary aspergillosis, and occupational asthma are syndromes representing pathologic changes in the bronchopulmonary system in response to the inhalation of environmental contaminants. In each syndrome, the inhalant
agent may have been contacted from occupational sources,
but such association is predominant, of course, in occupational asthma and hypersensitivity pneumonitis.
These conditions are relatively common, and estimates
as high as a 2% worldwide prevalence have been made.
Allergic bronchopulmonary aspergillosis is much less
common but must be considered in any patient with asthma
who develops signs of an acute bronchitis or pneumonitis.
     Each condition is associated with immunoreactivity
which may play a significant role in its pathogenesis.
Specific IgE antibodies are invariably present in ABPA
and present in the allergic forms of OA, while precipitating antibodies of the three major classes of immunoglobulins are closely correlated with episodes of ABPA,
HP and occasionally OA. Combinations of both immune
mechanisms, as well as cellular immune reactions and
complement activations have also been discovered in
these syndromes.
     The diagnoses are made by history, including relation to exposures, effect of change of environment, immunoserological and skin tests, and bronchial challenge
tests. Treatment has generally been rewarding when
irreversible changes such as bronchiectasis or interstial fibrosis have not developed. Control of these
conditions involves not only the proper care of the
individual patient, but industry-wide measures where
there is epidemilogical evidence of high prevalence.
Such measures require the cooperation of industry, unions, workers, and governmental agencies with health
and medical personnel. As more such cooperation is
forthcoming, it is likely that preventative measures
will result that should materially decrease the morbidity and mortality from occupationally related lung disease.

TABLE 4
Occupational Asthma: Precipitating Factors

Material	Industry or Trade
Ammonia, sulfur dioxide, hydrochloric acid, chlorine, nitrogen dioxide	Chemical and petroleum industry, silo fillers
Formalin	Medical
Animal, bird, fish, and insect-serum, dander, secretions	Veterinarians, animal and poultry breeders, laboratory workers, fishermen, sericulture
Castor bean, green coffee bean, papain, pancreatic extracts	Oil and food industry
Enzymes from *Bacillus subtillis*	Detergent industry
Hog trypsin, ethylene diamine, phthalic anhydride, trimellitic anhydride	Plastics, rubber, and resin industry
Phenylglycine acid chloride sulphone chloramides	Pharmaceutical industry
Complex salts of platinum	Metal refining
Salts of nickel	Metal plating
Flour, grain	Bakers, farmers, grain elevator operators
Wood dusts	Wood mills, carpenters
Vegetable gums (acacia, karaya)	Printers
Ampicillin, spiramycin, piperazine, amprolium hydrochloride	Pharmaceutical industry
Toluene diisocyanate	Polyurethane industry
Pyrolysis products of PVC price labels, plastic wrap	Meat wrappers
Soldering fluxes	Electrical trade

| Organic phosphorus insect-icides | Farm workers |
| Cotton dusts | Textile industry, vegetable oil |

REFERENCES

Reed, CE: Hypersensitivity pneumonitis, Postgraduate Medicine. 51:120-129, 1972.

Lopez, M, Salvaggio, J: Hypersensitivity pneumonitis: Current concepts of etiology and pathogenesis. Annual Review of Medicine. 27:453-463, 1976.

Pepys, J: Hypersensitivity diseases of the lungs due to fungi and organic dust. Basel: S. Kargin, 1969.

Hinson, K, Moon, AJ, Plummer, S: Bronchopulmonary aspergillosis, Thorax, 7:317-333, 1952.

Campbell, MJ, Clayton, YM: Bronchopulmonary aspergillosis: correlation of the clinical and laboratory findings in 272 patients. American Review of Respiratory Diseases, 89:186-196, 1964.

Rosenberg M, Patterson, R, Mintzer, R, et al: Clinical and immunologic criteria for the diagnosis of allergic bronchopulmonary aspergillosis. Annals of Internal Medicine, 86:405-414, 1977.

Murphy, RL Jr: Industrial diseases with asthma, In: Bronchial asthma, mechanisms and therapeutics. Boston: Little, Brown, & Co., 1977.

Pepys, J: Clinical and therapeutic significances of patterns of allergic reaction of the lungs to extrinsic agents, American Review of Respiratory Diseases, 116:573-588, 1977.

Slavin, R: Occupational asthma, Hospital Practice, 133-146, 1978.

Stephen R. Stewart
and M. Eric Gershwin

DEFENSE MECHANISMS OF THE LUNG

INTRODUCTION

The primary functions of the lung include gas exchange, acid/base balance, and specific certain metabolic processes. At rest a 60 kg man breathes approximately 7-8 L/min., of which 5L reaches the alveoli, where 300 ml of oxygen is absorbed and 250 ml of carbon dioxide expelled; thus accounting for only 5% of the inspired total. In addition to the passage of these large volumns of air, the lungs must carry out a number of secondary functions, including filtration of inhaled particulate matter of varying size and shape, process of various chemicals and toxins, and defense against ambient pathogens. Indeed extremely efficient barriers have developed against invasion of the organisms through the airways. These defense mechanisms can be divided into several categories, including mechanical, reflex, mucociliary, reticuloendothelial and immune.

MECHANICAL BARRIERS

Several factors influence the rate and site of particulate deposition. These include oral versus nasal inhalation; size, shape, density and charge of inhaled particles, flow velocity and airway aerodynamics. Particles of different sizes are deposited by different mechanisms. (Table 1) Particles less than 0.5 microns and greater than 10 microns in diameter are eliminated by filtration. The nasal fimbrai and turbinates are the initial filters, as well as being responsible for the removal of soluble gases including ozone, sulfur dioxide, and ammonium. Particles between 2 and 10 microns in size are largely deposited in the posterior pharynx by impaction. As the airstream changes direction in the oropharynx, mass and momentum

characteristics of these particles prevent their following the airstream and result in impaction against
the posterior pharyngeal wall. The tonsils and adenoids are concentrated at the sites of the greatest
density of particle deposition. The remaining particles are impacted at the carina or within the first
two bronchial divisions. Indeed approximately 90% of
10 micron particles and 20% of 2 micron particles are
deposited in this fashion. Particles from 5.0 down to
0.2 microns are generally deposited via sedimentation,
taking place in peripheral lung regions with low-flow
characteristics secondary to gravitational forces.
Particles smaller than 0.1 microns are largely deposited
via brownian motion resulting from their constant bombardment by gas molecules. Particles from 0.5 down to
0.1 microns are the least affected by inertia, gravity,
or brownian forces, and approximately 80% of particles
this size are exhaled.

TABLE 1

Deposition of Particulate Matter In The Lung

Particle Size	Mechanism	Site
>10 microns	Filtration	Nasal fimbrae
< 0.5 microns		Turbinates
2 - 10 microns	Impaction	Posterior oropharynx
0.2 - 5 microns	Sedimentation	Peripheral lung
>0.1 microns	Brownian Motion	Peripheral lung
0.05 - 0.1 microns	Exhaled	

Consideration of these physical characterictics is
not only of academic interest, and may be applied to
several clinical situations. For example, it has been
shown that pollen such as bluegrass, of 25 micrometer
diameter, only reach   the oropharynx; although a
large portion is swallowed, almost no intact pollen
particles reach the lung parenchyma. Asbestos, on the
other hand, which is 300 x 1 micron, exhibits special
aerodynamic characteristics which allow it to reach all
the way to the lung periphery. Similarly, morbidity
secondary to pulmonary edema from inhalation of aerosolized cooking fat can be avoided by changing the
particulate size and therefore altering the depth of
penetration. This is also a consideration in optimiz-
ing the delivery of various therapeutic pharmacologic

agents indluding inhalant steroids, cromolyn, and vasoactive substances into optimal areas of the lung.

REFLEXES

     Several reflex reactions are available for protect-
ion of the lung. Of prime importance is bronchoconstriction, a vagus-mediated smooth muscle contraction
accompanied by edema. Stimuli include mechanical irritation of the nose, trachea, or larynx, by irritant
gases, droplet aerosols, or inert dusts. The resulting increased resistance without change in compliance
allows severe constriction in airway calibre, while
maintaining peripheral air exchange units patent. The
great decrease in dead space thus protects from deep
penetration into the lung.
     The cough reflex is the major protection against
accumulated secretions and foreign material and results
in rapid expulsion. The physiology involved includes
deep inspiration, expiration against a closed glottis
thereby generating intrapleural pressures greater than
100 mm Hg. The glottis is then opened, resulting in
rapid reduction of bronchial calibre and greatly increased air flow rates up to 85% the speed of sound.
Secretions and foreign material may temporarily occlude
the lumen and then are propelled outward. In peripheral
areas of the lung with low-flow characteristics, cough
produces a milking action of the mucus transport system.
Some pathologic conditions such as chronic obstructive
pulmonary disease, emphysema, and cystic fibrosis may
result in ineffective cough with either retrograde or
cross aspiration of secretions and particulate matter
between the lungs. Increased viscosity and decreased
elasticity of secretions coupled with decreased compliance and increased resistance in the airways, prevent the appropriate mobilization.
     With regard to mucociliary transport, the cilia
beat in sequential metachronic transport waves at about
20 c.p.s. The origin of their pacer function is unknown. A progressive increase in the clearance rate
and velocity occurs from the peripheral to the central
airways. All particulate matter from a single inhalation will be eliminated within 24 hours. Derangements
in mucociliary transport are caused by several agents.

Cigarette smoke, sulfur dioxide, 100% oxygen, barbiturates, viruses, ethanol, and atropine all slow transport. Terbutaline and cholinergics increase the rate of transport.

RETICULOENDETHELIAL

The major cellular defense mechanism of the lung is the alveolar macrophage. This cell population has a wide range of scavenger-type functions which include physical removal of particles and dead cells, antigen processing in conjunction with T lymphocytes, bacterial removal in conjunction with antibody-complement mediated inflammatory responses, and activation for efficient pathogen removal in acute and chronic infection.

The macrophage originates in the bone marrow as an immature, nonactivated cell and then migrates to areas of inflammation. The migration of macrophages is slower than neutrophils and macrophages are a primary effector of cell-mediated immunity and delayed hypersensitivity reactions. Migration is modulated by lymphokines and other chemotactic factors liberated from lymphocytes primed by various antigenic substances. Lymphokines both attract and inhibit the egress of macrophages from areas of inflammation.

Macrophages have several exogenous and endogenous functions. They liberate a number of chemically active substances including plasmin inactivator, stimulation factors, collagenase, and lysozyme; these may enhance their ability to penetrate diseased parenchyma and concentrate at sites of damage. They also liberate chemotactic factors which attract other macrophages. Macrophages are capable of phagocytosis after which lysosomal contents are discharged into ingested vacuoles. Lysosomal contents hydrolyze bacterial membranes, enhance the effect of antigen-antibody-complement complexes, and interefere with bacterial metabolism through the liberation of toxic fatty acids and other substances.

Macrophages may become "activated" by interaction with primed regulator T cells to more efficiently perform a number of functions. (Table 2) T cells regulate activation by means of elaboration of lymphokines, migration inhibition factor, through stimulation of B cell antibody production. B cells produce antigen

specific antibodies and interact with macrophages via
antibody dependent cellular cytotoxicity. Activated
macrophages attain several functional characteristics,
including higher lysosomal content, enhanced phagocytosis, and enhanced bactericidal capacity. Both specific
and nonspecific enhancement has been demonstrated.
For example, activated macrophages are more efficient
killers of all bacteria, and may be specifically more
bactericidal for certain pathogens such as pneumococcus
during active infection with this organism. Macrophages rapidly lose their activation characteristics and
are depleted in numbers with resolution of specific
infections. There is no macrophage memory associated
with activation in the absence of lymphocyte interactions. The ability to activate macrophages may be
depressed by certain toxins and viruses.

TABLE 2
Features of Activated Macrophages
1. Higher lysosomal content
2. Enhanced phagocytosis
3. Enhanced bacteriocidal capacity
4. Elaboration of MIF
5. Antigen specific enhancement via antibody dependent
    cytotoxicity

IMMUNE SYSTEM

     Despite the efficacy of mechanical and cellular fac-
tors, substantial quantities of particles and solid
material reach the lung mucosal surfaces. The immune
system is largely responsible for processing and eliminating the remainder of these through several mechanisms.
Functionally, the immune system can be divided into
two major interrelated cell systems. Under local de-
velopmental influences multipotential stem cells differentiate into thymic derived or T cells with regulator and helper function, whereas bursa or B cells
attain immunoglobulin synthesizing capacity. (Figure 1)
Local mucosal immunity is primarily mediated through
production of an immunoglobulin, IgA. This primary
local immunoglobulin is present in high concentrations
in mucosal secretions and is the first line of defense
against inhaled antigens. IgA is produced locally by

DIFFERENTIATION OF THE CELLULAR IMMUNE SYSTEM

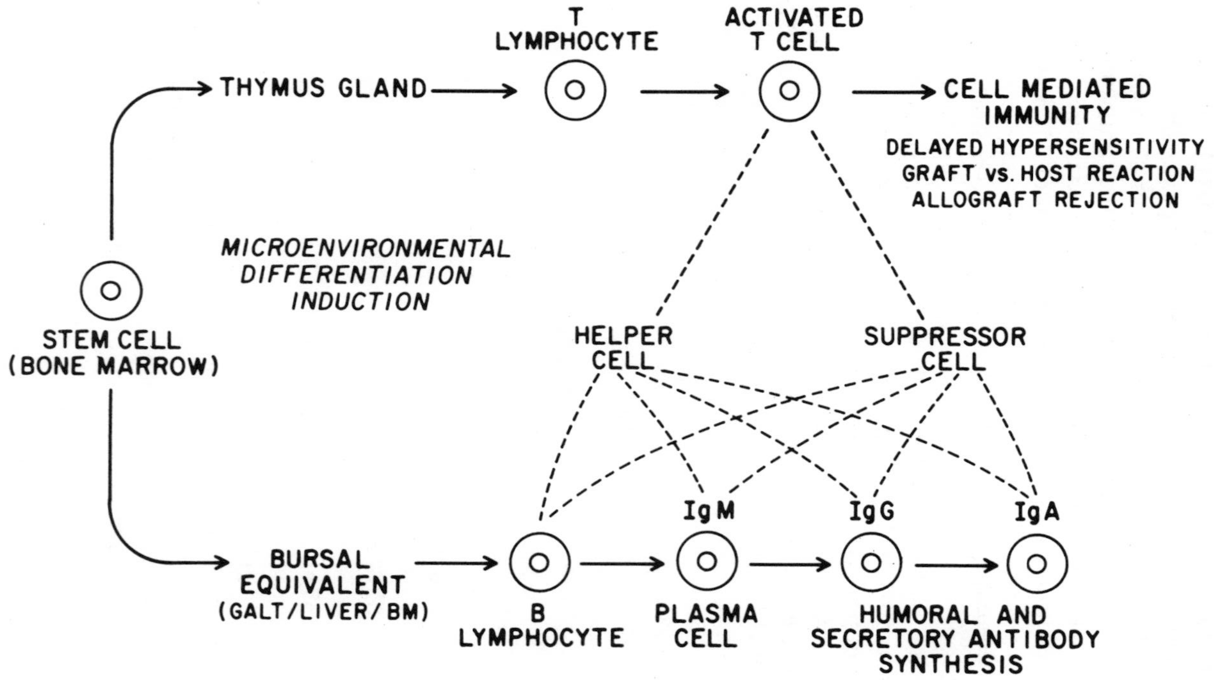

FIGURE 1

plasma cells in the lamina propria. It is secreted in
an 11S dimeric form and, within the apex of the pseudostratified columnar epithelial cells, is coupled to secretory component, a stabilizer which prevents proteolytic and enzymatic inactivation. (Figure 2) The stimulus for production of IgA is contact with local antigen. IgA is a non-complement fixing antibody with limited capacity for activation of the alternate pathway. (Table 3) It is, however, a strong agglutinizing
agent that can block viral or bacterial adherences to
cell surfaces and thus enhance elimination. By com-
bining with macromolecules, it can control absorption
and thus modulate the systemic immune response. IgA is
a local, short-lived antibody, with relatively limited
anamnestic response and blunted secondary responses as
compared with circulating IgG. It is proposed that plasma cell precursors are stimulated via T lymphocytes in
the bronchi-associated lymphoid tissue (see below) from
whence they circulate throughout the thoracic duct and
central circulation back to the parenchymal lamina propria, primed for local production of antigen specific
antibodies.

     Another important local antibody in the lung is
IgE. IgE is normally present in small quantities in
close proximity to the mucosal surfaces. A large portion is bound to surface receptors on mast cells. Although the primary function of IgE is unknown, it is
speculated to play an important role in response to
parasitic infestation. The IgE-mast cell system is
unique in that it contains tremendous capacity for am-
plification and production of physical responses. IgE
is a non-complement fixing antibody. (Table 3). Contact with antigen results in rapid mast cell degranulation with resultant immediate release of potent vasoactive amines which cause bronchospastic and local inflammatory reactions. In general, IgE is seen in high
concentrations in hypersensitivity and anaphylactoid
type reactions.

     Those substances which penetrate the local barriers
gain access to the systemic immune system. Recently,
study of the lymphoid system of the lung has demonstrated the existence of a bronchus-associated lymphoid
tissue (BALT). These special collections of lymphoid

follicles resemble Peyer's patches seen in the small
intestine. The overlying surface epithelia have special transport function which is thought to be important in antigen sampling. T cells are present in high
concentrations within these follicles and, probably
through interaction with antigen, macrophage, and B
cells regulate the production of the systemic immune
response. It appears that structural organization decreases as bronchial divisions progress peripherally.
Either by exposure due to loss of local mucosal integrity or absorption of soluble factors not removed by
IgA, the humoral systemic immune response can be elicited. Again, T cells are the regulator cells in this
response, inducing plasma cells to produce antigen
specific antibodies. The circulating antibodies are
the IgM and IgG classes and are capable of a much
higher degree of specificity and memory than the local
IgA system. (Table 3). They both are capable of activating complement and thus generating the inflammatory
response with resultant neutrophil chemotaxis, elaboration of vasoactive substances, enhanced opsonization,
and cytolysis. In addition to the circulating immune
system, lymphocytes are responsible for several cell-
ularly mediated immune responses. Certain antigens including some viruses, fungus, and other intercellular
pathogens induce cell-mediated immunity. Here again,
T cell acts as regulator for both macrophage activation,
direct cellular cytotoxicity by killer lymphocytes, and
non-specific cytotoxic reactions mediated by lymphokines.
The result is a delayed hypersensitivity reaction.

     After exposure to an antigenic substance, several
types of immunopathologic responses can be elicited.
The immediate or hypersensitivity reaction is the type
seen in allergic phenomena. This pathologic response
is IgE mediated and may result in intense local or
acute systemic reactions. These range clinically from
urticaria-angioedema to bronchoconstriction with asthma
and anaphylactic shock. These reactions are more commonly seen in atopic (perhaps genetically predisposed)
individuals to a variety of antigens including dust,
pollen, molds, and chemicals. The humoral antibody
system activation results in a subacute response. This
is an antibody, antigen, and complement mediated res-

ponse that results in induction of inflammation. The antibody may be specific for a pathogen, i.e. pneumococcal
pneumonia; a cross reacting lung autoantibody, i.e.,
Goodpasture's syndrome; or nonspecific, i.e., the circulating DNA-anti DNA- complement complexes seen in
lupus pulmonary vasculitis. This process results clinically in pulmonary infiltrative lesions and vasculitis with hemoptysis. The other major type of immunopathologic response is delayed hypersensitivity. These
are generally classified as lymphocytotoxic reactions
that result in direct and kinin related cytoxotocity,
macrophage activation, and granuloma formation. Here
again, these reactions may be antigen specific, such
as TB granuloma, or (possibly) nonspecific, i.e.,
Wegner's granulomatosis or sarcoidosis. Finally,
there are mixed reactions which may, depending upon
the antigens and complexity of the induced response result from a combination of any or all of the above
mechanisms. Several disease processes have been im-
plicated to have multiple immunopathologic origins.
These include the demonstration of cytotoxicity,
hypersensitivity pneumonitis and granulomatous pulmonary vasculitis, and IgE plus antigen-antibody-complement reactions to Aspergillus antigens in allergic alveolitis.

It is important to keep in mind the concept that
the lung defense system is a dynamic equilibrium between the mechanical, reflex, cellular, and local and
systemic immune mediated responses. The functional
integrity of the system also depends upon a complex
interaction between the host, the antigen, and the
environment. Several factors are known to modulate immune responses in the lung. (Table 4). The genetic
background of individuals may determine the class and
quantitative response of the immune system to certain
antigens. This is dramatically demonstrated in the
recent outbreak of coccidioidomycosis in California,
with major increases in susceptibility demonstrated in
patients with Negro and Philippino ethnic origins. In
addition, it is possible that abnormal responses to certain antigens may predispose to underlying pathologic
conditions such as the apical bolus emphysema and fibrosis seen in ankylosing spondylitis. In addition to
inherited considerations, several factors in relation

to the antigenic exposure will influence the immune re-
ponse. The dosage, time interval, route of administration, and previous sensitivity to an antigen may pro-
foundly influence the type, quantity, and course of the
immune reaction. A number of antigenic interactions
may take place which influence the response, such as
viral induced immune supression predisposing to bacterial infection, or the enhanced oncogenesis of the as-
bestos-smoking combination. The underlying state of
the host, including age, sex, nutritional and emotional
status, concomitant systemic or chronic illness and
previous antigenic exposure may also influence the
immune response. The integrity of the regulatory and
processing system is also critical.

TABLE 4
Factors Modulating Pulmonary Immune Responses

Host	Genetic Predispositions
	Emotional and Nutritional States
	Age and Sex
	Concomitant Systemic or Chronic Illness
	Immuno Deficiency States
	Drugs
Antigen	Dosage
	Time Interval
	Route of Administration
	Previous contact with Ag
	Contact with Other Ags
	Drugs

IgA and immunoglobulin deficiencies can be shown to
predispose the individual to recurrent pulmonary infection, chronic obstructive, lung disease, bronchiectasis, and asthma, as well as a variety of autoimmune
phenomenon. Cell mediated immune deficiencies result
in increased susceptibility to fungal and certain viral
pathogens, as well a possible reduced oncogenic sur-
veillance and resultant increased incidence of lymphoma and neoplasias.

The continuous bombardment of the nasopharyngeal
and pulmonary tree by potential pathogenic stimuli has
led to highly sophisticated mechanical, reflex, cellular,
and immune defense mechanisms for their elimination.

TABLE 3
Properties of Immunoglobulins

Property	Classification of Immunoglobulin				
	IgG (γG)	IgA (γA)	IgM (γM)	IgD (γD)	IgE (γE)
Normal serum concentraion mg/100 ml (±1 SD)	1,240 (±220)	390 (±90)	120 (±35)	3 (±3)	0.05
% of total serum immunoglobulin	70 to 80	10 to 15	5 to 10	0.2 to 1	0.002
Molecular weight	160,000	170,000– 385,000	900,000	180,000	200,000
Biologic function	Principal serum anti- body	Secretory antibodies	First antibody formed in re- ponse to antigen	Unknown	Anaphylactic reactions
Primary distribution	Extracellular fluid	External secretion (tears, saliva, intestinal juices,	Intravascular	Intravas- cular	Reaginic antibody

colostrum)

Biologic half-life (days)	23	5.8	5.1	2.8	2.3
Fractional catabolic rate (% of intravascular pool catabolized per day)	6.7	25	18	37	89
Synthetic rate (mg/kg/day)	33	24	6.7	0.4	0.02

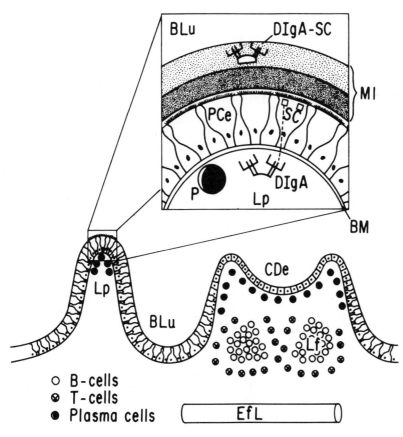

BRONCHUS ASSOCIATED LYMPHOID TISSUE
AND IgA SECRETION

FIGURE 2

Lp-Lamina propria; BLu-Bronchial lumen; CDe-Cuboidal
Dome epithelium; Lf-Lymphoid follicle; EfL-Efferent
Lymphatic.   Insert: P-Plasma cell; DIgA-Dimeric IgA;
PCe-Pseudostratified Columnar epithelium; SC-Secretory
Component; Ml-Mucin layer.

Even subtle derangements in these systems or their interactions may doom a patient to recurrent infection,
asthma, early chronic lung disease or neoplasia. Enhancement of responses to bacterial pathogens with antibiotics or replacement of immunoglobulin deficiencies
with gammaglobulin are current examples of ways physicians can alter the consequences of inadequate defense
mechanisms. Future study into the underlying mechanisms for these derangements will undoubtedly expand
our armamentarium for altering the clinical consequences.

REFERENCES

Dannenberg AM: Macrophages in inflammation and infec-
    tion. NEJM 293: 489, 1975.
Fishman AJ, Pietra GG: Handling of bioactive materials
    by the lung, I and II. NEJM 291: pp 884-890 and
    pp 953-960 1974.
Kaltreider HB: Expression of immune mechanisms in the
    lung. Am Rev Resp Dis 113: 347 1976.
Newhouse M, Sanchis J, Bienenstock J: Lung defense
    mechanisms I and II. NEJM 295: pp 990-998 and
    pp 1045- 1052 1976.
Podheski WK: Autodestructive mechanisms provoked by
    lymphocytes. Am J Med 61:1 1976.
Rosenow GC: The spectrum of drug induced pulmonary
    disease. Am Int Med 77: 997 1972.
Schatz M, Patterson R, Gink J: Immunopathogenesis of
    hypersensitivity pneumonitis. J All Clin Immunol
    60: 27. 1977.
Tomasi TB: Secretory immunoglobulins. NEJM 287: 500
    1972.
Wilson AF, Novey HS, Beshe RA, Surprenant, EL: Deposi-
    tion of inhaled pollen and pollen extract in
    human airways. NEJM 288: 1956 1973.

Ralph C. Frates, Jr.

TWO CHRONIC PULMONARY SYNDROMES OF CHILDHOOD: CYSTIC
FIBROSIS AND GASTROESOPHAGEAL REFLUX WITH ASPIRATION

INTRODUCTION

Two of the most common causes of serious and recurrent pulmonary disease in children are cystic fibrosis
and gastroesophageal reflux with aspiration. These
two clinical entities should be considered strongly in
the differential diagnosis of the child with significant respiratory complaints. All too often, however,
the patient with either of these syndromes is mistakenly labelled an "asthmatic" or "an allergic child."
Failure to recognize these disorders is especially re-
grettable since both treatment and prognosis of cystic
fibrosis and of gastroesophageal reflux are different
from asthma, and delay in diagnosis adversely affects
outcome.

CYSTIC FIBROSIS—GENERAL COMMENTS

The first of these syndromes, cystic fibrosis or CF,
is a chronic progressive disease of genetic origin
which affects infants, children, adolescents and even
adults. The customary or textbook picture is that of
a child with chronic bronchitis with marked cough, pancreatic exocrine insufficiency with malabsorption, steatorrhea, and greatly increased concentrations of sodium
and chloride in sweat. However, the more that is known
about cystic fibrosis, the more clinical variation in
expression of the gene is appreciated.
While the cause of cystic fibrosis remains almost as
obscure as when "cystic fibrosis of the pancreas" was
first described by Fanconi in 1936 and by Anderson in
1938, it is still true that the exocrine glands are the
recognized target organs. While understanding of the
role of mucin in pathogenesis of this disease is still
not certain, the mucus-secreting glands and cells of

153

the respiratory, digestive, and reproductive tracts
seem to be responsible for obstructive damage to these
systems. On the other hand, serous secretions from
the parotid, submaxillary, and eccrine sweat glands
are mainly notable for abnormal electrolyte concentrations.

CF is apparently an autosomal recessive disease and
the most common serious genetic disorder among Caucas-
ians, with generally quoted incidence of 1 in 2000
live white births. The disease is much rarer among
blacks than among whites and rarer still among Orient-
als with most of these cases reported within the United
States. It should be noted, however, that the pattern
of genetic inheritance of cystic fibrosis is open to
question. Indeed it has been proposed that CF is determined by two dominant alleles located at two autosomal
loci, with interaction between these loci.

RESPIRATORY COMPLICATIONS OF CYSTIC FIBROSIS

Of particular concern to the practitioner are the
respiratory complications of cystic fibrosis. In an
anatomical sense, the respiratory complications of CF
begin with nasal polyps. These growths are common,
allegedly occurring in up to 20% of patients, and may
be the first recognized sign of CF if not confused with
allergic nasal polyps. They may remain asymptomatic,
obstruct the nasal passages to the degree that they
cause mouth-breathing, and/or produce pansinusitis with
postnasal drip. Indeed the literature notes that
polyps may become mucocoeles and generate bone erosion.
Treatment of symptomatic polyps is surgical excision,
although they frequently recur. Of far greater clinical significance than nasal passages associated with
morbidity and mortality in CF, are lower airway involvement: at least 90% of CF patients die because
of chronic lung disease. Exactly when the lungs become abnormal is uncertain. Microscopic examination
of the lungs of CF neonates dying of meconium ileus
are reportedly unremarkable. Soon, however, the pathologic picture changes to chronic bronchiolitis with
hypertrophied mucus glands and cells, followed by mucus
plugging, chronic infection, and bronchorrhea. Results
of sophisticated serial pulmonary function tests such

as helium-oxygen flow volume loop determinations concur
with the pathological evidence: airway obstruction begins in the bronchioles, then advances to major airways.
  Overwhelming *Staphylococcus aureus* bronchopneumonia
with septicemia, commonly a presenting picture of
cystic fibrosis in infancy during the pre-antibiotic
era, is now rarely seen. Antibiotic therapy localizes
the infection long enough to permit the host to build
high specific antibody titers to the common bacterial
respiratory pathogens of CF, with resultant chronic
bronchitis and bronchiectasis. The reasons for selection of these specific bacterial pathogens remains
unknown. In the natural history of CF, *Staphylococcus
aureus* is the predominant cause of infection, while
Haemophilus influenza, E. coli, proteus and other organisms are less commonly cultured from sputum. In
more recent years, however, *Psuedomonas aeruginosa,*
particularly the characteristic and peculiar mucoid
strain, has emerged as the organism most often recover-
ed from sputum cultures. Presumably, aggressive antibiotic therapy has played a role in the changing bacterial population of the CF patients' airways. That is,
Staphylococcus aureus and *Hemophilus influenza* are
either eradicated or suppressed by antibiotics to the
point where *Psuedomonas aeruginosa* moves into those
organisms' ecological niche.
  Symptomatically, infections are first manifest as a
persistent cough. Over periods of time varying from
weeks to decades the patient develops other symptoms
of chronic bronchitis. These symptoms include wheezing
and production of purulent sputum. This latter symptom
may be invisible to parent and practitioner at first,
since infants and children often swallow rather than
cough out sputum. An astute questioner will ask the
parents if they have felt or heard the child's chest
"rattling," as a sign of purulent mucus in the airways.
As the obstruction of airways progresses, the cough becomes more violent and often productive of green or
yellow sputum, the chest diameter increases abnormally;
diffuse rhonchi and rales are heard on auscultation.
Digital clubbing is ever-present, probably representing
lung tissue destruction. The patient is poorly nour-
ished with diminished muscle mass and often a protuber-
ant abdomen. Exercise tolerance is limited. A chest

roentgenogram will reveal hyperinflated lungs with varying degrees of interstitial fibrosis, atelectasis, in-
filtrate or even bronchiectasis. Even now the patient
and parents may be told the diagnosis is "asthma!"

TREATMENT OF CYSTIC FIBROSIS

Proper treatment rests on early diagnosis. The *sine
qua non* of cystic fibrosis are repeatedly elevated
sweat chloride concentrations obtained by quantitative
pilocarpine iontophoresis technique. The positive
sweat test must be in combination with any one of the
following criteria: chronic pulmonary disease, pancreatic insufficiency, or a family history of CF.

Treatment of the respiratory complications of CF is
surprisingly similar to the program for an adult patient with any chronic obstructive lung disease except
-to some degree- in the selection and use of antibiotic
agents. Great emphasis is placed on bronchial hygiene,
since many or even most CF patients suffer from a voluminous bronchorrhea unusual in other forms of chronic
bronchitis. Chest percussion and bronchial drainage
with inhalation of various bronchodilators are commonly
prescribed on a twice-daily basis and more often when
needed. Patients should be kept fully immunized, including annual influenza vaccination with the current
vaccine. There is no uniformly agreed-upon therapy for
massive hemoptysis or for recurrent pneumothorax: many
authors advise bronchoscopy with an eye toward pulmonary resection or *in situ* vascular occlusion for the
former, and chest tube placement with intrapleural in-
stillation of sclerosing agent for the latter. Recently, however, the Cleveland CF Center has reported good
results by treating patients with massive hemoptysis
with transfusions, antibiotics, postural drainage and
vitamin K administration. Many CF patients given aggressive treatment aimed at controlling bronchitis, including low-flow oxygen, diuretics, and sometimes di-
goxin, have gone on to enjoy a few additional years of
quality life.

Bronchial lavage has also been advocated in the
treatment of CF. The purpose of the lavage is to remove mucoid impactions in the bronchi and bronchioles
and in so doing, improve ventilation and gas exchange.

Different centers have advocated alternative techniques
including rigid bronchoscopy under general anesthetic,
fiberoptic flexible bronchoscopy with lavage in alert
patients, and even drowning one lung at a time with
liters of fluid via the patient's tracheal tube. Although there are claims to the contrary, clinical data
does not decisively show lessened morbidity or mortality in patients so treated versus a more conventional
approach to therapy.

More surprising than the lack of agreement among
different CF Centers on the value of bronchoscopy or
low-flowing oxygen therapy is the disparity in the way
in which antibiotics are prescribed. There are no well-
controlled long-term studies proving that taking an antibiotic or antibiotics on a daily basis lessens bronchitic symptoms or delays death. Many physicians now
prescribe antibiotics only when the patient shows signs
of exacerbated respiratory infection, including more
frequent and productive cough, weight loss, less able
performance on simple tests of pulmonary function
(i.e. peak expiratory flow rate) and dyspnea. The
chest film may remain unchanged and the patient a-
febrile throughout many such episodes. As for choice
of antibiotic, there are several good semisynthetic
penicillinase-resistant drugs for treatment of staphylo-
coccal infection. Psuedomonas infections, however, are
currently amenable to treatment with only a few antibiotics. Against the psuedomonas, the physician most
often will depend on intravenous carbenicillin or ti-
carcillin and hope for synergy with an aminoglycoside
such as gentamicin or tobramycin. Standard oral antibiotics (i.e. tetracycline) are increasingly ineffective against psuedomonas with two outstanding exceptions: trimethoprim-sulfmethoxazole and chlorampheni-
col. In the experience of many clinicians, chloramphen-
icol works even when sensitivity studies indicate that
the drug should be useless. As a general rule of
thumb, antibiotic therapy for bacterial respiratory
"flare-ups" in a CF patient should be in high doses
for at least two weeks.

Finally, it is important to discuss the results of
all this tremendously expensive and time-consuming
effort. Again, there are no control populations for
comparison, but the average life span of the cystic

fibrosis patient followed in a CF Center has increased
from about a dozen years a decade or more ago to the
threshold of adulthood today. Most of this increase
in lifespan is not because of the diagnosis of large
numbers of CF patients at later ages; furthermore as
important as the length of life is the quality of that
life. A number of recent surveys illustrate the fact
that many if not all patients remain in sufficient
psycho-social harmony with the world to complete their
educational goals, marry, and get on with life in general until there is very little life to live. Compas-
sionate and knowledgeable physicians and other profes-
sionals and lay persons can do a great deal to help
make the CF person's life worthwhile.

GASTROESOPHAGEAL REFLEX WITH ASPIRATION

Gastroesphageal reflex (GER) with aspiration has
only been appreciated as a cause of recurrent pulmonary disease in children for the last decade. The major
reason for this late appreciation of the awareness of
the nature and magnitude of GER-related pediatric lung
disease is the lack of diagnostic techniques beyond
the routine esophagram. Use of newer techniques, including esophageal manometry with perfused catheters,
intraluminal pH probe for acid reflux, and the flexible
fiberoptic pediatric endoscope, are responsible for understanding the physiology of the lower esophageal
sphincter.

Prior to this understanding, older terminology sub-
stituted for correct knowledge of physiology with the
expected confusing results. For example, throughout
voluminous medical writing, hiatus hernia was thought
to be a major cause of aspiration. Similarly, chala-
sia, or cardioesophageal relaxation was reported to
be benign and expected in infancy. In fact achalasia,
or esophageal distension from an overly "tight" esophageal sphincter, was frequently treated with dilatation or esophageal myotomy alone. There were, however,
a smattering of excellent but isolated reports in the
American Pediatric literature of radiographically "silent" regurgitation resulting in lung injury or destruction but these reports were generally ignored by
most specialists and practitioners alike.

In 1971, Cohen and Harris, using a manometer with a
perfused catheter, clearly demonstrated that in adults
the symptoms of GER (heartburn and regurgitation) correlated with a lower esophageal sphincter pressure
(LESP) of 10 mm of mercury or less. Hiatus hernia had
no effect on gastroesophageal sphincter competence.
This study called to question the rationale for hiatal
hernia surgery and moved the problem of reflux from
surgical to medical and then to pediatric attention.
Since 1971, there has been a rapid increase in the
number and pertinence of papers on GER with aspiration.
Danus *et al* in 1976 were among the first to focus interest on the incidence of GER with aspiration in children. Choosing in a random fashion 43 infants and
young children with "recurrent obstructive bronchitis"
seen at a pulmonary outpatient clinic 26 infants showed varying degrees of reflux on esophagrams. All
these infants and 17 other bronchitic infants and
children without roentgenographically proven reflux
had LESPs lower than age-appropriate controls. Most
of these patients gained weight and improved symptomatically with medical therapy for reflux. It is important to note that the patients of Danus *et al* had
"... minimal to absent" gastrointestinal symptoms and
no characteristic chest x-ray changes.

It is now apparent that although the incidence of
GER with aspiration is not precisely known, this syndrome is probably a common but occult variety of pulmonary disorder in children as well as adults. In one
of the largest series published to date, Fonkalsrud
and co-workers, reinforced and extended the new concept of GER with spillage as a cause of lung disease.
Their report summarizes their experience at UCLA in
patients from 2 weeks to 19 years of age undergoing
Nissen fondoplication for GER. The duration of their
study was 9 years. From that series a number of important points can be made (Table 1).

TABLE 1
Symptoms of GER

Symptom	Number
Repeated emesis	56/74
Failure to thrive	20/74
Pneumonia or recurrent	18/74

respiratory infections

Dysphagia due to stricture	12/74
Dysphagia due to achalasia	4/74
Asthma	5/74
Epigastric	4/74

Of particular interest in this study is the impression of the relative efficiency of the different diagnostic procedures (Table 2).

TABLE 2
Diagnostic tests for GER

Test	% positive
Thin barium esophagram	78
Tuttle test (pH reflux)	85
Esophageal manometry (LESP 14 mmHg)	66
Esophagoscopy:	
Gross and microscopic esophagitis	15
Microscopic esophagitis with normal gross	20
Esophageal stricture	16

With respect to diagnosis, however, these and other authors note the "limited accuracy" of the esophagram, relegating this procedure to a screening role. Even with this intensive approach to diagnosis, 6 infants with allegedly repeatedly symptomatic GER had all normal studies but greatly improved after surgery. Finally, it is worth noting that the authors concluded all of their 74 patients undergoing Nissen fondoplication were cured or greatly improved without a single death or serious complication.

What can a practitioner faced with a coughing, wheezing baby or child do? First, the physician must consider the diagnosis of GER with aspiration. His or her index of suspicion of GER with aspiration must be very high in those patients for whom there is no obvious explanation for their worsening condition on adequate therapy, or in those patients who have a prediliction for occult aspiration (i.e. cerebral palsy patients, Down's syndrome children, Sandifer's syndrome, postoperative tracheoesophageal fistula repair patients.) Second, the practioner should look further into signs or symptoms of GER such as vomiting, failure to thrive,

and anemia. Even in patients with possible pulmonary
complications of GER who have no GI symptoms, an esophagram may prove worthwhile. If the esophagram shows
spontaneous reflux to or above the carina, the chance
of GER with aspiration being an explanation for pulmonary symptoms is great. At this point, a trial of medical therapy is worthwhile in the less sick aspiration patients.

TREATMENT OF GER

   Carré has outlined an often-effective program.
Babies 6 months or younger can be seated upright in an
infant chair around the clock and fed formula thickened with cereal. Children have the head of their bed
or crib raised 60° or 8 inches from the floor on blocks
and are fed nothing after dinner. Antacids are helpful
if esophagitis symptoms are present. The outlook for
this group of GER patients seems quite good: Carré
and his colleagues report most infants treated in this
manner stop vomiting by 12 months of age. Furthermore,
over 90% of their patients were symptom-free 20 years
later. However, Lilly and Randolph reported the failure of medical therapy in 9 out of 9 of their patients
2 years of age or older. Given this information, the
practitioner should attempt medical therapy with confi-
dence in infants but with skepticism in older children.
   The sicker patients, however, should probably be referred to a pediatric gastroenterologist at a tertiary
care center. The aggressive UCLA group recommends a
trial of medical therapy for 6 weeks before a decision
is made on surgery. In their opinion, those patients
with proven esophageal strictures and severe failure-
to-thrive infants should promptly go to the operating
theater once a diagnosis of GER is established. Their
choice of procedure is the Nissen fondoplication, in
which the stomach is freed up, then plicated around
the intra-abdominal esophagus. This group's excellent
results have already been mentioned in this article.

FUTURE DIRECTIONS IN GER

   A final note... there are as yet many unanswered
questions about the prevalence, diagnosis, and treat-

ment of GER. For example, there has yet been no large
number of childhood asthmatics studied using the current means available with an eye toward definition of
the role of GER in that disease. The indications for
surgery are imperfect. Medication such as bethanecol
may eventually become the therapy of choice for mild
reflux. Early reports suggest the 24 hour pH probe
may possibly better define significant reflux than do
present methods. With physicians becoming more aware
of reflux resulting in pediatric pulmonary disease,
the evolution of superior diagnostic means and criteria
and of improved treatment should progress rapidly.

REFERENCES

Anderson, D.H.: Cystic fibrosis of the pancreas and
    its relation to celiac disease: A clinical and
    pathological study. Am J Dis Child 56: 344, 1938.
di Sant' Agnese P. A., Davis, P.B.: Research in cystic
    fibrosis. N Engl J Med 295: 481, 534, 597, 1976.
Luck, S.R., Raffensperger, J.G., Sullivan, H.J., et al:
    Management of pneumothorax in children with chronic
    pulmonary disease. J Thoracic and Vasc Surg 74: 834,
    1977.
Wood, R.E., Boat, T.F., Doershuk, C.F.: Cystic fibro-
    sis: state of the art. Am Rev Resp Dis 113: 833,
    1976.
Waring, W.W.: Current management of cystic fibrosis. In
    Advances in Pediatrics. Edited by L.A. Barnes, Year
    Book Medical Publishers, 1976, 401.
Euler, A.R., Ament, M.E.: Value of esophageal manome-
    tric studies in gastroesophageal reflux of infancy.
    Pediatrics 59: 58, 1977.
Euler, A.R., Ament, M.E.: Detection of gastroesophageal
    reflux in the pediatric age patient by esophageal
    intraluminal pH probe measurement (Tuttle test).
    Pediatrics 60: 65, 1977.
Danus, O. Casar, C., Larrain, A., Pope, C.E.II: Eso-
    phageal reflux--an unrecognized cause of recurrent
    obstructive bronchitis in children. J Pediatr 89:
    220, 1976.
Fonkalsrud, E.W., Ament, M.E., Byrne, W.J., Rachelefsky
    G.S.: Gastroesophageal fondoplication for the man-
    nagement of reflux in infants and children. J

Thorac Cardiovasc Surg 76: 655, 1978.

Carré, I.J., Astley, R., Langmead-Smith, R.: A 20-year followup of children with a partial thoracic stomach (hiatal hernia). Aust Paediatr J 12: 92, 1976.

Lilly, R.R., Randolph, J.G.: Hiatal hernia and gastro-esophageal reflux in infants and children. J Thorac Cardiovas Surg 55: 42, 1968.

Glen A. Lillington

PULMONARY ASPIRATION SYNDROMES

INTRODUCTION

The anatomical "crossover" of the respiratory and gastro-intestinal tracts at the laryngeal-hypopharyngeal level creates the potential for aspiration - the entry of liquids or solid particles through the glottis into the tracheobronchial tree and even into the peripheral air spaces. The clinical syndromes resulting from aspiration will depend upon the amount of material aspirated, the relative solidity or liquidity of the aspirate, the chemical properties of the aspirate, the presence or absence of pathogenic micro-organisms, and the extent of involvement of the lung parenchyma. Wheezing is a common symptom, and this may lead to an incorrect diagnosis of "asthma" if the occurrence of aspiration is not recognized.

PROTECTION AGAINST ASPIRATION

Swallowing (deglutition) is a complex coordinated neuromuscular manuever which accomplishes the transfer of solid or liquid foodstuffs from the oropharynx to the hypopharynx-esophagus while preventing entry into the tracheobronchial tree. This mechanism may be impaired by any one of a number of diseases or abnormalities, including:

1) diseases causing muscular weakness of the larynx or pharynx, such as bulbar palsy, poliomyelitis, muscular dystrophy, myasthenia gravis and others.

2) diseases causing anatomical alterations of the larynx or pharynx.

3) the presence of endotracheal tubes or a tracheostomy, which mechanically interfere with swallowing.

4.   Obtundation

The larynx acts as the "watchdog of the lungs,"
responding with violent coughing and laryngospasm to
the presence of foreign material in or near the glottis.
This protective mechanism, constantly present, is inde-
pendent of the swallowing reflex, but may be impaired
under certain circumstances:

1) certain materials, including mineral oil and
the normal pharyngeal secretions, are relatively non-
irritating and, in small quantities, can slip through
the glottis without arousing a defensive response

2) the presence of an endotracheal tube within the
glottis holds the vocal cords apart and permits free
aspiration of hypopharyngeal liquids

3) obtunded states decrease the sensitivity of the
laryngeal reflexes and facilitate aspiration, particularly if the hypopharyngeal area is flooded, as by
vomitus. Such states include general anesthesia,
alcoholic obtundation, sedative drug overdosage and
even normal sleep.

ASPIRATION SYNDROMES

The term "aspiration pneumonia" is nonspecific
and its use tends to mask the profound differences in
etiology, pathogenesis, clinical manifestations and
choice of therapy between the different disease states
which result from aspiration. The entry of foreign
material into the respiratory tract may give rise to
one or more of at least six different syndromes
(Table I). Pneumonic consolidation does not invariably
occur, and when present, may be associated with widely
varying pathological and clinical manifestations.
Bilateral wheezing occurs in approximately one-
third of patients with peptic pneumonitis but the
extensive radiological abnormalities provide clear
evidence that the patient does not have asthma.
Roentgenographic changes may be mild or absent in the
patients whose wheezing is due to foreign body aspiration or to recurrent minor aspirations of gastric juice
secondary to hiatal hernia.

TABLE I
Aspiration Syndromes

Syndromes	Pathogenesis
The cafe-coronary	Glottic impaction
Tracheobronchial foreign bodies	Aspiration of solids
Peptic pneumonitis	Aspiration of gastric acid
Chronic or recurrent regurgitant lung disease	Pharyngo-esophageal disorders
Lipid granuloma of lung	Aspiration of fats or oils
Necrotizing pneumonia	Aspiration of infected secretions

THE CAFE-CORONARY (FOOD CHOKING)

The impaction of large bolus of solid food within
the glottis may lead to asphyxia and a rapid demise.
In some cases, the true cause of the catastrophe is
not recognized at the time, and the supposition that
the individual has succumed to an acute exacerbation
of heart disease has given rise to the term "cafe-
coronary."

An excess of preprandial cocktails is an important
contributory factor in many instances. The offending
substance is often incompletely masticated beefsteak.
The typical clinical presentation is for the diner,
who is aphonic, to clutch his throat or to gesticulate
wildly and point to his mouth. Cyanosis develops
rapidly but may be undetectable in the subdued illumi-
nation of many restaurants. An unrelieved complete
obstruction causes collapse and death within a few
minutes.

The diagnosis must be made promptly and treatment
instituted rapidly to avert catastrophe. Although
pounding the victim's back while holding him upside
down is often effective in children, it is technically
difficult in the adult. In rare instances, an emergency tracheotomy, with improvised surgical tools, has
been performed successfully (within 3-5 minutes) on
the asphyxiating patient lying on a restaurant floor,
but this can hardly be recommended as standard therapy.

It seems reasonable for the bystander to make one
attempt to dislodge the impacted food bolus by hooking
a finger through the mouth into the victim's hypo-

pharynx. If this is unsuccessful, the Heimlich maneuver should be employed. Although complications may occur, this technique is frequently successful. It has recently been suggested (Guildner) that compression of the lower chest has a higher success rate than the Heimlich maneuver and is less traumatic. As the Heimlich maneuver can be self-applied, the life you save may be your own.

TRACHEOBRONCHIAL FOREIGN BODIES

Particulate solid objects which may enter the tracheobronchial tree include bones, pins, nuts, tacks, teeth, dental drills, coins and virtually any small object, which for one reason or other, a person may put in his mouth.

In the past, foreign body aspiration has mainly occurred in small children, but this problem has diminished a little with the realization by parents that peanuts are not ideal foodstuff and that small objects less than 1 cm in diameter (such as beads) are not well suited for playthings. A growing problem is the "handyman" who holds nails or tacks in his mouth while working. Facial trauma results in a perennial crop of aspirated tooth fragments; the trauma may include the sudden application of a fist or a windshield to the face, or the detachment of teeth by overvigorous larnygoscopy.

The clinical picture resulting from aspiration of a foreign body is variable. Paroxymal coughing or choking occurs immediately after aspiration but may subside quickly. The infant or young child cannot relate this information and if the aspiration occurs when there is no older observer in the vicinity, the diagnosis may be missed. In many cases, there is an asymptomatic "silent" interval which may last moments, hours, days or years. If the silent interval is prolonged, even the adult may fail to associate his present pulmonary symptoms to the past episode of choking,

In some cases, such as peanut aspiration, the foreign body evokes a violent chemical reaction in the bronchial mucosa. In most instances, the foreign body is inert and the lung disease results from mechanical obstruction of the bronchus. Abnormalities may include

obstructive hyperinflation, atelectasis, bronchiectasis,
recurrent pneumonia, and lung abscess. Occasionally
the patient may be asymptomatic for years. Wheezing
respirations simulating asthma may be present. This
type of "asthma" responds poorly to standard therapy
but may be quickly relieved by removal of the foreign
body. Wheezing may be bilateral even though the foreign
body is unilateral.

The diagnosis is easily established if the foreign
body is radio-opaque. If the article is radio-lucent,
radiological evidence of partial or complete bronchial
obstruction should be sought. If the chest roentgenogram shows one lung to be relatively "black" (hyper-
lucent) and the other lung to be "white (opaque), it
may be difficult to decide whether the patient has
obstructive hyperinflation in the black lung or obstructive atelectasis in the white lung. Comparison of
end-inspiratory and end-expiratory chest films is helpful in this differentiation. As only the unobstructed
lung can show significant volume change during respiration, the mediastinum will appear to shift towards the
normal lung on expiration (actually it is the chest
wall on the unobstructed side which moves toward the
mediastinum).

Bronchoscopic removal of the foreign body is the
treatment of choice and is almost always successful.
The rigid bronchoscope has a wide lumen which facilitates the passage and manipulation of instruments.
In a few cases, the fiberoptic bronchoscope has been
employed successfully. In an occasional instance,
thoractomy with bronchotomy is necessary.

PEPTIC PNEUMONITIS (MENDELSON SYNDROME)

This castastrophic syndrome is an acute bilateral
alveolar-filling process secondary to the aspiration
of large quantities of gastric juice of low pH. Patho-
logically it is actually a hemorrhagic pulmonary edema
of chemical origin. The pH of the aspirated fluid
must be less than 2.5 to produce the syndrome.

The commonest cause is the administration of
general anesthesia, particularly for obstetrical or
emergency surgical procedures. Other predisposing
factors include comatose states, convulsive disorders

and the passage or presence of nasogastric or gastric
lavage tubes.

The pulmonary reaction develops rapidly and presents radiologically as a diffuse alveolar consolidation, usually bilateral, and often perihilar in distribution. Differentiation from cardiogenic pulmonary
edema is aided by the normal heart size and the absence
of signs of pulmonary venous hypertension (such as
Kerley "B" lines and cephalad redistribution of blood
flow). The pulmonary capillary "wedge" pressure is
normal. All of these features, of course, occur in
any type of noncardiogenic pulmonary edema and are not
peculiar to peptic pneumonitis. This emphasizes the
importance of a documented history of vomiting with
aspiration. Atypical radiological localizations may
be noted.

Symptoms and signs develop rapidly, usually within
an hour of the aspiration. These patients are obviously seriously ill, with dyspnea, cyanosis, fever, cough,
tachypnea and (often) wheezy respiration. Functionally,
the lungs are small and stiff, with hypoxemia so severe
that even high concentrations of inhaled oxygen may
fail to relieve it - i.e. the patient has "adult respiratory distress syndrome."

If the occurrence of aspiration is suspected but
cannot be confirmed from the history, bronchoscopic
demonstration of diffuse segmental and subsegmental
bronchial erythema may be diagnostically helpful, as
this phenomenon is not a feature of noncardiogenic
pulmonary edema unless aspiration or influenza are the
causative factors. The specificity of this finding is
completely lost if the patient has been intubated for
some time and has developed a bronchial superinfection.

Treatment must be prompt and vigorous. If the
aspiration occurs in the operating room, bronchoscopy
to remove food particles and any excess vomitus is
warranted, but attempts to lavage the bronchial tree
or neutralize the fluid with bicarbonate solution are
of questionable value. Adrenal corticosterids are
commonly employed although recent studies have cast
doubt on the efficacy of this treatment and some
studies suggest it may do more harm than good. A
beneficial effect is more likely if the steroid is
given early--within an hour after aspiration--and

discontinued after 24-48 hours.

Proper management of the hemorrhagic pulmonary edema is of the utmost importance. The edema is due to increased capillary permeability and will show little response to diuretics and none to digitalis. Therapy should include the following:

1) bronchodilators if wheezing is present

2) serial blood gas measurements to monitor therapy

3) oxygen supplementation to keep PaO$_2$ above 60

4) intubation and mechanical ventilation if oxygen alone (with FIO$_2$ of 0.5 or less) fails to keep PaO$_2$ above 50. PEEP may be required.

Antibiotics are useful only if secondary infection occurs in the later stages of the disease. Such nosocomial infections are common in intubated patients and difficult to treat.

CHRONIC AND RECURRENT REGURGITANT LUNG DISEASE

Patients with esophageal disorders frequently have recurrent episodes of regurgitation and aspiration of retained esophageal or gastric contents. As the aspirated material is often small in volume and the pH is usually not too low, the pulmonary reactions are less violent. Although each episode may be clinically mild, the recurrent nature of the disorder may eventually result in extensive permanent lung damage.

The syndrome was first described in cases of achalasia (cardiospasm), but it may also occur with Zenker's diverticulum, hiatal hernia, esophageal strictures, neuromuscular disorders of deglutition, and tracheoesophageal fistulas.

Bronchopulmonary abnormalities which may result include chronic cough, bronchiectasis, localized pulmonary fibrosis, chronic wheezing and recurrent pneumonias. The pneumonias may involve different areas of lung at different times, and are often physicochemical in nature rather than infectious.

Esophageal regurgitation due to hiatal hernia is a rare but important cause of chronic "intrinsic"

asthma. Appropriate medical or surgical therapy for
the hernia may alleviate or relieve the wheezing
attacks.

LIPID PNEUMONIA

Aspiration of animal and vegetable fats (in food)
usually causes an acute pneumonic reaction. In contrast, mineral oil is relatively bland; it can pass
through the glottis with little if any cough, and
results in a low grade chronic granulomatous process
in the dependent area of the lung. Radiologically it
appears as a segmental consolidation or peripheral mass
which simulates bronchogenic carcinoma, and is known as
a paraffinoma.
The diagnosis can be suspected if a history of
mineral oil use is obtained, but biopsy confirmation
is essential in most instances. The presence of lipo-
phages in sputum is not specific enough for the diagnostician to conclude confidently that carcinoma has
been excluded.

NECROTIZING PNEUMONIA

The aspiration of infected oropharyngeal secretions may cause an acute bacterial pneumonia with necro-
sis and lung abscess formation. Common predisposing
factors include peridontal infections, alcoholism,
comatose states, convulsive episodes and deglutitional
disorders. Inhalation of blood or tissue fragments
during tonsillectomy, sinus operations or dental procedures was an important cause in the past but is now
mainly of historical interest.
In community-acquired infections, the offending
bacterial are usually anaerobes, as these organisms are
the major components of the normal oropharyngeal flora.
Hospitalized patients frequently have pharngeal colonization by staphylococci or aerobic gram-negative
bacilli, and nosocomial aspiration pneumonias are
often caused by these organisms, which, like the anaerobes, are often necrotizing. Previous antibiotic use
also promotes colonization.
Lung abscess secondary to anaerobic aspiration
pneumonia is often called "primary" lung abscess,

although the term "postpneumonic" is clearly more
appropriate. Other terms that have been employed include "putrid lung abscess" and "gangrene of the lung."
Empyema is also a common complication of necrotizing
pneumonias.

Clinical features include high fever, cough, leucocytosis in peripheral blood and physical signs of consolidation (in many cases). With rupture of the abscess
into a bronchus, copious amounts of purulent sputum,
often foul smelling, appear. Hemoptysis is common.
Radiologically, the pneumonitis-abscess initially
appears as a segmental consolidation or peripheral mass;
with rupture and drainage, the typical air-filled thick
walled cavity is apparent, often with a horizontal
"fluid level."

Differential diagnosis should include bronchial
obstruction causing obstructive abscess, loculated
pyopneumothorax, cavitating lung tumor, tuberculosis,
fungal infections, infected lung cyst, amebiasis, sep-
tic infarction and collagen diseases (such as Wegener's
granulomatosis). Bronchoscopy should be performed (at
least once) for the following reasons: 1) to rule out
bronchial obstruction (tumor, foreign body), 2) to
obtain material for cultures, and 3) to help establish
or improve drainage.

REFERENCES

Abjulmajid OA et al: Aspirated foreign bodies in the
    tracheobronchial tree: report of 25 cases. Thorax
    31: 635, 1976.
Andersen HA et al: Pulmonary complications of cardio-
    spasm. JAMA 151: 608, 1953.
Bartlett JG et al: The bacteriology of aspiration pneu-
    monia. Am J Med 56: 202, 1974.
Genereux GP: Lipids in the lung: radiologic-pathologic
    correlation. J Can Assoc Radiol 21: 1, 1970.
Guildner CW, Quoted by Stephenson HE: Cardiopulmonary
    resuscitation. Chapter 37 in Respiratory Care,
    J.B. Lippincott, Philadelphia, 1977.
Heimlich HJ et al: Food-choking and drowning deaths
    prevented by external subdiaphragmatic compression.
    Ann Thorac Surg20: 188, 1975.

Huxley EJ et al: Pharyngeal aspiration in normal adults
and patients with depressed consciousness. Am J
Med 64: 564, 1978.

Iverson LIG, May IA, Sampson PC: Pulmonary complications in benign esophageal disease. Am J Surg 126:
223, 1973.

Landay MJ, Christensen EE, Bynum LJ: Pulmonary manifestations of acute aspiration of gastric contents.
Am J Roentgenol 131: 587, 1978.

Lillington GA et al: Removal of endobronchial foreign
body by fiberoptic bronchoscopy. Am Rev Resp Dis
113: 387, 1976.

Mackowiax PA et al: Pharyngeal colonization by gram-
negative bacilli in aspiration-prone persons.
Arch Int Med 138: 1224, 1978.

Peterman AF, Lillington GA, Jamplis RW: Progressive
muscular dystrophy with ptosis and dysphagia.
Arch Neurol 10: 38, 1964.

Ruggers G, Taylor G: Pulmonary aspiration in anesthesia. West J Med 125: 411, 1976.

Wolfe JE, Bone RC, Ruth WE: Diagnosis of gastric aspiration by fiberoptic bronchoscopy. Chest 70: 458,
1976.

Wolfe JE, Bone RC, Ruth WE: Effects of corticosteroids
in the treatment of patients with gastric aspiration. Am J Med 63: 719, 1977.

Paul J. Donald

NASAL POLYPOSIS

INTRODUCTION

The finding of polyps in the nasal cavities is a not too uncommon occurrence. By far the commonest type is the so-called allergic polyp, commonly seen in patients with allergic rhinitis. Since polyps and infection go hand in hand, many of these patients suffer from chronic rhinosinusitis as well. The management of patients suffering from this disorder is one of the greatest challenges put to the otolaryngologist.

CLASSIFICATION

Although the nasal polyps found with the highest frequency are allergic in type, many other polyps of diverse origins exist as well. Accurate identification is essential; the inadvertent biopsy of a lesion such as a juvenile nasopharyngeal angiofibroma that has been mistaken for an innocuous polyp will surely treat the attendant physician to a sanguinous surprise. Unfortunately, many intranasal soft tissue masses look alike. Some form of classification (Table 1) is necessary in order to make proper distinctions that will guide appropriate therapy.

The allergic polyp is an outpouching of mucosa that is pedicled on a relatively narrow stalk (Figure 1). The peeled grape appearance possessing a greyish or an off-whitish hue is characteristic. It is covered by attenuated respiratory epithelium, and its stroma is made up of sparse connective tissue, much edema fluid, many eosinophils, some neutrophils, and a few lymphocytes. They hang in the nasal cavity pedicled on the middle meatus, the middle turbinate, and occasionaly on the septum. The mucosa of the rest of the nasal cavity is frequently a pale, bluish color with a boggy appearance. There is often an attendant clear or

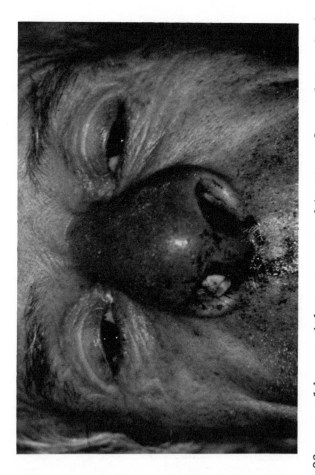

FIGURE 1: An 82-year-old man with a two-year history of total nasal obstruction and periodic epistaxis due to nasal polyposis. Excision via ethmoidectomy gave complete relief.

purulent rhinorrhea. The polyps are insensitive to palpation with a suction tip and do not bleed on such contact. They are very soft and freely mobile.

TABLE 1
Classification of Nasal Polyps
A. Benign
    1. Congenital
        a. Encephalocele
        b. Glioma
        c. Dermoid
    2. Allergic
    3. Inflammatory
    4. Neoplastic
        a. Squamous Papilloma
        b. Juvenile Nasopharyngeal Angiofibroma
B. Malignant
    1. Inverting Papilloma
    2. Esthesioneuroblastoma
    3. Squamous Cell Carcinoma
    4. Adenocarcinoma
    5. Malignant Melanoma
    6. Sarcoma
    7. Metastatic

    The inflammatory polyp is beefy red, sensitive to
touch, and bleeds easily. It is often bathed in mucopus, and its pedicle is broad. The consistency is
firm, and the polyp is less mobile than those due to
allergy. Microscopically the lesion demonstrates a-
bundant fibrous tissue and many capillaries with numerous neutrophils as well as collections of lymphocytes.
This polyp is really much like a granuloma in that it
is a response to chronic infection. In chronic rhinosinusitis, inflammatory and allergic polyps are often
found side by side.
    Congenital nasal masses are rare. Heterotrophic
brain tissue may be found in the nasal cavity presenting as a firm, mucosally covered polyp. This results
from a failure of the neural tube to adequately separate itself from the primitive nasal ectoderm during
embryogenesis. If the central connection of the mass
is through suture lines at the skull base, the mass
will present in the nasopharynx. If the dural connec-

tion is through the cribriform plate, the lesion presents in the nose and/or externally. The anteriorly located ones often present with hypertelorism, nasal obstruction, and epiphora. In those patients in whom continuity with the subarachnoid space remains intact, the mass will pulsate and be seen to swell as the child cries or if the ipsilateral internal jugular vein is occluded by digital pressure. When an encephalocele becomes pinched off from the rest of the central nervous system, the neural elements degenerate or take on a bizarre appearance. The glial and fibrous elements predominate. A child with such a lesion is differentiated from one with an encephalocele in continuity with cerebrospinal fluid by the lack of pulsation or swelling with increasing cerebrospinal fluid pressure. This lesion is commonly known as a "nasal glioma". The danger of intranasal biopsy of either of these lesions is a cerebrospinal leak or meningitis. Tomography of the skull base will often delineate the point of connection between the encephalocele and the brain.

Intranasal dermoids originate as inclusion cysts in the midline of the nose. They can occur anywhere from the glabella to the nasal tip. Very frequently they connect with the suture lines between the nasal bones and the adjacent frontal bone or maxilla. These embryonic inclusion cysts commonly present as a swelling in the region of the root of the nose, but occasionally an intranasal component will appear as a polyp. A pit in the midline of the nose with hairs protruding from it and an underlying mass are pathognomonic of this lesion.

Benign neoplastic lesions are very uncommon but are important to recognize. The juvenile nasopharyngeal angiofibroma is a benign tumor composed of numerous blood vessels in a dense, fibrous tissue stroma. It is found principally in preadolescent males. Although the tumor takes origin in the clivus and grows into the nasopharynx, it may only become initially apparent as a polypoid nasal mass. A portion of its purplish appearance and rock-hard consistency may be obscured by the polypoid degeneration and pale appearance of the overlying mucosa (Figure 2). This lesion is extremely hemorrhagic and biopsy usually produces a massive hemorrhage.

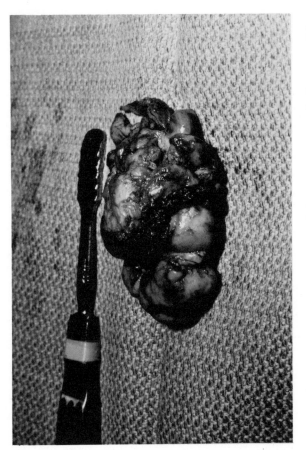

FIGURE 2: Juvenile nasopharyngeal angiofibroma removed from a 14-year-old boy.

The squamous papilloma is a polypoid pink growth of fibrous tissue covered by normal mucosa. It is soft and resembles the surrounding mucosa. Of itself it is of little importance, but its relative, the inverting papilloma, is an entirely different matter.

The malignant tumors are divided according to those that are more characterized by local aggressive growth in contrast to those that spread by discontinuity and metastasize. Although the inverting papilloma never metastasizes, it is characterized by exuberant local invasion. Its appearance is grossly indistinguishable from its benign counterpart, the squamous papilloma. Radiographically, the maxillary and even ethmoidal sinuses may be opacified often with evidence of adjacent bone destruction. Biopsy reveals the characteristic endophytic papillary configuration of the lesion as it erodes into adjacent tissues. Adequate therapy can only be employed by radical excision with at least a 2 cm margin of healthy tissue around the periphery of the lesion.

Esthesioneuroblastoma is a rare tumor originating in the olefactory epithelium. This explains its origin in the cribriform area and the superior meatus of the nose. It, like the inverting papilloma, is indistinguishable from the squamous papilloma on gross examination, although occasionally it is a deeper purplish hue. It is locally aggressive and, if originating on the cribriform area, requires a combined craniofacial excision. Local recurrence and direct spread into the anterior cranial fossa are unfortunately common. Metastases are uncommon (less than 20 percent) with the most usual sites being the cervical lymph nodes and lung.

Carcinomas in the nasal cavities are either primary or secondary. The commonest tumors to metastasize to this site are hypernephroma and malignant melanoma. The common primary tumors are squamous cell carcinoma and adenocarcinoma. Although a few may present as polypoid, mucosally-covered polyps, many are ulcerative and bleeding. In contrast to the benign polyps which usually present only with symptoms of nasal obstruction and rhinorrhea, the malignant lesions will, in addition, often complain of epistaxis and pain. Most malignancies presenting in the nasal cavities do not originate

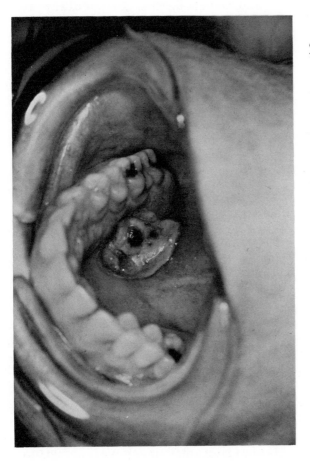

FIGURE 3: Adenocystic carcinoma of the maxillary sinus in a 48-year-old female presenting as a mass in the palate.

there but are extensions of primaries in the paranasal
sinuses. If the lesion takes origin in the maxillary
sinus, palatal swelling, the fairly rapid appearance
of an ill-fitting denture, or a swelling in the cheek
may be the presenting features observed.   Proptosis
signifies orbital invasion of tumor from either the
maxillary or ethmoidal sinuses and is a sign of far
advanced disease. The commonest early sign of both of
these tumors is epistaxis. The mass is usually very
hard to palpation and often bathed in purulent secretions. Since most of these neoplasms originate in the
maxillary or ethmoid sinuses, x-ray examination often
shows bone destruction in the lateral wall of the nose
as well as the other walls of the affected sinuses.
Diagnosis is made on biopsy of the lesion in the nose
and exploration of the affected sinuses to delineate
the extent of tumor. The most effective treatment is
a combination of radiotherapy and radical excision.

CHRONIC SINUSITIS

     Nasal polypsis is commonly found in association
with chronic inflammatory disease of the paranasal
sinuses. The polyps are often a mixture of inflammatory and allergic types with the latter predominating.
In the normal condition the mucosa lining the sinuses
possesses a mucous blanket which is continuously propelled by cilia in the direction of the sinus ostia.
When infection supervenes, the cilia become deactivated.
Secretions stagnate and putrefy, producing a yellowish
or greenish, thick, foul-smelling material known as
"mucopus." The presence of polypoid mucosa obstructs
the ostia, further impeding the egress of purulent
secretions.
     Acute sinusitis is a relatively easy diagnosis to
make. The presence of acute pain over the maxillary
antra, behind the eyes, or over the forehead coupled
with fever, nasal obstruction, and purulent rhinorrhea
are clear signs of this disorder. Radiographic evidence of sinus opacity establishes the diagnosis.
     Chronic sinusitis is more occult. Often the only
complaint is purulent postnasal discharge. Pain is a
less common symptom while nasal obstruction is much
more common, especially in the presence of nasal poly-

posis. A history of allergic symptomatology is frequently elicited. Seasonal or perennial allergic
rhinitis sets the stage for the development of polyposis
and subsequent sinusitis. Examination may show merely
the presence of polyps. Often spraying with a vaso-
constrictor, such as Neo-synephrine or cocaine 2%, is
necessary to shrink the mucosa sufficiently to demonstrate the presence of mucopus. Tenderness is occasionally found over the affected sinus involvement.
Ethmoidal tenderness is perceived when pressure is
applied over the area of the lamina papyracea on the
medial wall of the orbits. Frontal tenderness is best
elicited by palpation of the inferomedial aspect of the
orbital roof or by tapping across the medial aspect of
the forehead. Radiographic examination in the Cald-
well, Waters, submentovertical, and lateral projections
is an invaluable aid in making the diagnosis.

Many patients go through life with nasal obstruction and postnasal discharge ignorant of the fact they
have a time bomb in their heads ready to explode at any
time. These explosions are complications, many of
which have serious, even fatal, consequences. Since
the advent of antibiotics, osteomyelitis of the bone
surrounding the infected sinus cavity is uncommon. Despite this fact, patients with this complication are
regularly seen in the large ear, nose, and throat de-
partments across the country. The commonest bone affected is the frontal bone. Meningitis, subdural abscess, cerebritis, and brain abscess can occur from
the direct spread of infection or via retrograde thrombophlebitis in the small venula connecting sinus lumina
to the extradural veins. The most disastrous complication is cavernous sinus thrombosis (Figure 4). This
condition, with its characteristic toxicity, high
fever, proptosis, chemosis, and frozen globes, carries
a 50 percent mortality despite vigorous therapy with
modern antimicrobials. Cavernous sinus thrombosis is
important to distinguish from orbital cellulitis and
orbital abscess. The latter two conditions are more
common and usually result as a direct extension from an
ethmoidal sinusitis. The unilateral nature of these
inflammatory disorders of the orbit coupled with the
lack of profound toxicity that usually accompanies
cavernous sinus thrombophlebitis help to make the diag-

184

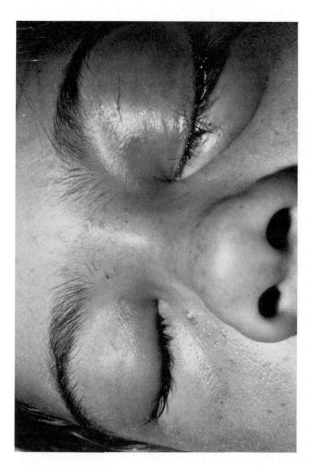

FIGURE 4: Cavernous sinus thrombosis in a 14-year-old boy. Disease was secondary to an acute ethmoid sinusitis.

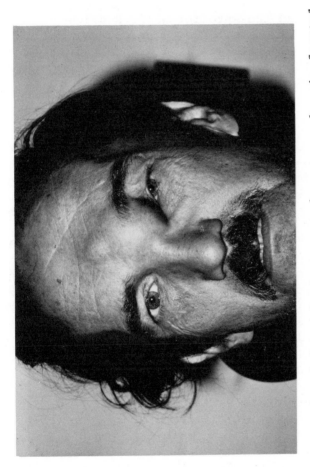

FIGURE 5: Mucopycele of frontal sinus secondary to a chronic frontal sinusitis.

nosis.

The frontal sinus is peculiarly vulnerable to a
rather unusual complication. If its ostium is obstructed by chronic sinusitis, polypoid mucosa, or a fracture secondary to trauma, the mucosa encysts and se-
cretes mucous into its lumen. This cyst or mucocele
takes on a bone erosive quality often penetrating one
or more of the walls of the frontal sinus. If it
erodes through the floor, the eye is pushed inferolater-
ally; if through the anterior wall, a subcutaneous cyst
is felt; and, if posterior erosion occurs, the intra-
cranial cavity is entered. The mucocele often becomes
infected (Figure 5). This mucopyocele, if intracran-
ial, can result in meningitis or a brain abscess.

TREATMENT

The bulwark of therapy for chronic sinusitis rests
on two prongs--management of the allergic diathesis
and eradication of the infection. A careful allergic
history is taken, and, if the slightest suspicion of
atopy is raised, the patient is skin tested. Desensitization is routinely employed in those cases that are
skin-test positive for inhalant allergens. There are
some physicians who will attempt a dust desensitization program even in the absence of a positive skin
reaction. Although the author does not advocate this
practice, it is not an uncommon stance that is taken
in the management of an otherwise extremely refractory
patient. A history of food allergy is sought, and pro-
vocatove testing employed if indicated. The skin
tests for food allergy and cytotoxic food testing procedures remain without adequate scientific foundation
to support them at this time.

The management of infection often requires a combined chemotherapeutic and surgical attack. The appropriate antibiotic should be established by culture
and sensitivity testing. Although culture results
differ in various geographic areas, most of the flora
are responsive to the administration of ampicillin.
A wide variety of decongestant-antihistaminic combinations are presently on the market. The selection of
the most appropriate of these agents is purely a trial-

and-error procedure on the part of the patient. Effective nasal mucosal shrinkage coupled with minimal side
effects are the goals striven for.

In the presence of polyps, desensitization, antibiotics, and antihistaminic-decongestant combinations
are often unsuccessful in the elimination of disease.
The injection of polyps with steroids, a once popular
and occasionally efficacious maneuver, has been discontinued because of the reported cases of blindness
following these injections. Topical steroid application, such as Decadron-Turbinaire, or the oral-adminis-
tration of Prednisone over a short period are sometimes successful.

The polyps then require some sort of surgical removal to ensure sinus drainage as well as open the airway. Polyps may be excised with a snare as an office
procedure. This is a temporizing measure giving temporary relief of nasal obstruction. When good allergic
control and appropriate antibiotic treatment follow,
this will occasionally give prolonged symptomatic relief. Unfortunately this is not usually the case.
Since most polyps take their origin in the maxillary
or ethmoidal sinuses, surgical intervention is usually
mandated. For maxillary sinus disease, the Caldwell-
Luc approach is commonly the procedure of choice.
Under local anesthesia, a gingival-buccal incision is
made through to the bone. The soft tissue is dissected
up to the infraorbital nerve, and a window is made in
the face of the maxilla. The entire mucosal lining of
the sinus complete with polyps is dissected and cur-
etted away. An antromeatal window is created through
the lateral nasal wall that is flush with the floor of
the nasal cavity. Occasionally a huge polyp will fill
the sinus, go through the sinus ostium, and present in
the nasopharynx. This antrochoanal polyp usually
takes origin on the lateral maxillary wall and requires
the Caldwell-Luc operation for successful removal.

When polyps originate in the ethmoid sinuses, an
ethmoidectomy is indicated. The intranasal ethmoidectomy is a highly successful but difficult operation to
perform. It can be done under local anesthesia through
the nose obviating an external excision. However, a
more thorough removal of the ethmoid block can be done
through external incisions made in the nasojugal area.

Direct visualization of the ethmoid block facilitates
safe and complete removal. The ethmoid cells, once
exenterated, leave a marsupialized bony cavity which
rapidly relines with epithelium.

The frontal sinus is best managed by total excision through an osteoplastic flap of the frontal bone
overlying the sinus. Obliteration of the sinus with
abdominal wall fat following complete mucosal excision
using a rotating burr results in complete ablation of
the sinus cavity. This is the most efficacious of all
the frontal sinus procedures with a failure rate of
less than 5 percent.

REFERENCES

Batsakis, J.G.: Tumors of the head and neck. Williams
    and Wilkins Co., Baltimore, Maryland, First Edition,
    pp 250-253, 1975.
Proctor, B., Proctor, C.: Congenital lesions of the
    head and neck. Otolaryngol Clin North Am 3(2): 244-
    245, 1970.
Hardy, J.M., Montgomery, W.W.: Osteoplastic frontal
    sinusotomy: An analysis of 250 operations. Ann
    Otol Rhinol Laryngol 85:523-532, 1976.

Stephen M. Nagy, Jr.
and Michael A. Klass

TREATMENT AND EVALUATION OF ACUTE AND CHRONIC
URTICARIA

INTRODUCTION

Urticaria, in its diffuse form, is extremely common. Indeed more than 20% of the population suffer
from it at some point during their lifetime. Moreover
for many such patients it persists as a terribly disabling and frustrating disorder. Urticaria, much like asthma, represents a final common pathway, an abnormal
reaction pattern, with multiple triggering factors and
diverse mechanisms and mediators. Many physicians mistakenly attributed urticaria to stress, emotion and the
litany of psychiatric diagnosis. Similarly urticaria
has lacked the glamour of a well defined clinical entity secondary to enzyme deficiency, genetic defect, or
abnormal protein; the "pot of gold" for the academic
researcher. Finally there is also perplexity for the
clinician dedicated to divisions and classifications
based on purest terms. The following review attempts
to follow a clinical sequence for urticaria, including
presentation, laboratory evaluation and treatment.

CLINICAL CHARACTERISTICS

The classic pathology of urticaria consists of pruritic, distinct, erythematous, elevated lesions that
blanch with pressure; they are not difficult to recognize. Usually such lesions are evanescent; wheals blo-
ssom dramatically only to fade in 20-30 minutes and re-
appear elsewhere. The size range of lesions includes
pinpoint (2-3 mm) to larger to giant wheals which may
coalese into non-erythematous areas of significant
swelling, i.e. angio-edema. Indeed urticaria is the
major clinical sign in hereditary angio-edema (HAE) a
well defined syndrome of a deficient component of com-

plement. In contrast angio-edema when it occurs in
"allergic" reactions tends to be less pruritic than its
idiopathic urticarial counterpart, more frequently involves the face, and is more likely to be associated
with gut and laryngeal involvement, manifested by
cramping abdominal pain and hoarseness.

Given the appropriate circumstances (i.e. an injection of penicillin, or a bee sting) the physician can
make the diagnosis by history. In fact, if the reaction is self-limited, this may be the only basis to establish a hyper-sensitivity state. On the other hand,
treatment and evaluation of an ongoing process is difficult until the actual lesions are observed. In
cases where lesions are recurrent but absent on the
initial office visit, the patient should be encouraged
to return with active lesions at any time. A significant minority will be found to have other dermatopathic
processes. Moreover a number of treatable, but potentially fatal systemic disorders present simply as severe pruritus and associated excoriations. Such patients are convinced that the lesions are spontaneous
(they scratch severely during sleep) and are not self-
induced. Polycythemia vera, Hodgkins disease, hypercal-
cemia and uremia, hepatic disease (especially biliary
cirrhosis) and scabies are all major etiologic considerations. The last dermatologic condition is characterized by terribly intense nocturnal pruritus and
the classical lesions may be totally obliterated.

Confusion may occur with other members of "vascular"
skin reactions. Toxic erythema consists of erythematous macules which may coalesce to form large areas of
involvement. Classical urticaria may be altered by
high dose antihistamine therapy, particularly hydroxyzine, and also present as macular lesions. Erythema
multiforme may be indistinguishable from urticaria, however, the lesions are usually more violaceous rather
than pink, are serepiginous, more symmetrical and clear
with a residual pigmentation. "Iris" lesions are typical, particularly on the hands and the feet. The elevated lesion of severe "vasculitis" does not blanch
with pressure and is associated with petechiae, ecchy-
mosis and ulceration. Although there is an initial
urticarial component in an insect bite, the non-evanes-
cent and indurated character of the delayed response

should obviate the differentiation. A host of other
skin diseases such as psoriasis, eczema, pityriasis
rosea and even early forms of bullous disorders (i.e.
dermatitis herpetiformis and pemphigus) may initially
resemble an urticarial eruption. In questionable
cases, the opinion of, and biopsy, by a dermatologist
is preferred.

PATHOLOGY

Histopathology of urticaria reveals dilation of
venules and capillaries, flattening of rete pegs, and
swollen appearing collagen bundles within the dermis;
edema is variable but may be considerable; cellular
infiltration is minimal with occasional neutrophils,
eosinophils, lymphocytes and histiocytes. Deposition
of immune complexes on or about the basement membrane
with variably low serum complement occurs in approximately 15% of chronically afflicted urticaria patients.
Whether this represents simply an abnormal response or
chronic antigenic stimulus is not clear. The changes
in angio-edema are quite similar, however, the edema
extends to the subcutaneous tissue. Unlike the more
severe end of the spectrum of the "vascular reaction"
group, epidermolysis, extensive perivascular infiltration and red cell exudation are not present.

MEDIATORS

There is a large body of evidence, both direct and
indirect, that histamine is a major mediator of the
urticarial response. Intradermal injection clearly re-
produces the wheal and especially the itching; antihistamines are also clinically effective in a large majority of afflicted patients; various immunologic and non-
immunologic (non-antigen mediated) reactions elicit
histamine release. There are a variety of mechanisms
by which histamine and other mediators are generated.
These include:
    1. The combination of antigen with IgE antibody
        bound to the basophil or tissue mast cell.
    2. Classical antigen--antibody reactions activat-
        ing the complement system. Components C3a and
        C5a interact directly with the cell surface to

    trigger histamine release.
3. Complement pathway activated directly at C3.
4. Direct release of histamine, without antibody
    or complement, by various drugs such as mor-
    phine, codeine, colymycin, curare, pentamadine,
    dextran, constituents of berries, especially
    strawberries, and possibly iodinated dyes.
    Kinins, prostaglandins, SRS-A, and serotonin share
various pharmacological properties with histamine, i.e.
    all have some effect on the microvasculature and in-
crease permeability. Beyond this their exact role in
urticaria is undefined and they are discussed more completely on pages 13-22.

HISTORICAL EVALUATION

    A major reason for distinguishing between an acute
self-limited episode and the chronic, recurrent form
of urticaria is practicality. If the diagnosis is by
history or the patient simply curious, then a limited
search for extrinsic etiology, (i.e. transfusions,
stings, drugs, and particularly allergenic foods) is
appropriate. Further investigation is then unwarranted.
In the acute stage, the physician must bear in mind
that urticaria is a common manifestation of anaphylaxis.
Autopsy cases have shown the mechanism of death to be
laryngeal edema in the majority. Therefore, the history should note voice change, hoarseness, "tickle in
the throat," clearing the throat, cough, or chest
tightness, all of which indicate possible laryngeal and/
or bronchial involvement. Inspiratory stridor with retraction indicate a markedly compromised airway and/
or intubation and tracheotomy strongly indicated. Such
life-threatening episodes demand a meticulous outline of
of exposures, especially foods, in the previous twenty-
four hours.
    The vast majority of acute cases clear within twenty
twenty-four to seventy-two hours. In the remainder,
whealing persists for one to two weeks and, for some, it
it does not cease. Six to eight weeks duration is the
current prerequisite for the designation "chronic."
Although such patients are usually non-atopic and have
a poorer prognosis for eventual clearing, the terminology instructs us less about the disease and more of

the physician's role. The "wait and see" attitude,i.e.
symptomatic management, of an apparently benign
self-limited disorder must evolve into a more aggressive and immaginative approach. Chapter 2 of this volume outlines the major historical considerations of
the allergic history. The review of systems should be
exhaustive and the physical examination complete and
thorough. The present illness, particularly if leng-
thy, can be tedious with patients attempting to describe in detail multiple episodes and their "inklings"
as to a precipitating cause. Although some idea as to
frequency should be recorded, neither that nor intensity give any clue as to etiology. The distribution
and character of the lesions are sometimes helpful.
The important specific questions, of course, are pre-
dicated on a full understanding of precipitating
causes.

ETIOLOGY

An operational classification is found in Table I.
The distinction between immunological and non-immunological is based on the presence in the former of
either elevated levels of a normal immunoglobulin (i.e.
IgE) or an abnormal protein, (i.e. cryoglobulin). With
the exception of HAE, immunochemical techniques offer
little help in the diagnosis of the latter which in the
great majority, is based on clinical presentation.

DRUGS

Immunologic reactions to drugs may be defined as
immediate, i.e. anaphylactic, occurring from within
three to twenty minutes, accelerated, from twenty minutes to forty-eight hours, and delayed, after forty-
eight hours. Skin involvement is common with all types
with urticaria and/or angio-edema occurring exclusively
in anaphylaxis and predominating in early accelerated
reactions while maculo-papular eruptions are more frequent in late accelerated and delayed responses. These
criteria were originally proposed to organize reactions
to penicillin based on the presumably responsible immunoglobulin. Our understanding has undergone some
change since that time, however, these criteria are

still clinically useful.

TABLE 1
Acute and Chronic Urticaria
Classification
Immunological

1) Drugs - IgE mediated except serum sickness (IgG).
2) Foods - IgE
3) Parasitic infestations - IgE
4) Inhalants (dander, pollens, wheat, fish) - IgE
5) Insect stings and bites - IgE
6) Transfusion reaction
7) Cryoglobulinemia - IgG, IgM
8) Cryofibrinogenemia
9) Collagen - Vascular disease
10) Cold hemolysin syndrome (syphilis - IgG)
11) Infectious illnesses (infectious hepatitis, infectious mononucleosis)
12) Hyperthyroidism
13) Urticaria pigmentosa
14) Contact - IgE

Non-Immunological

1) Drugs - histamine liberators, ASA and related anti-inflammatory compounds, iodinated dyes (mechanism unclear)
2) Hereditary angioedema
3) Foods - histamine liberators
4) Cold
   a) Familial
   b) Essential
5) Light - immediate and specific spectrum
6) Heat - very rare
7) Dermatographism
8) Cholinergic
9) Urticaria pigmentosa
10) Circinate urticarias
11) Stress

Anaphylaxis describes a syndrome characterized by broncho-constriction, laryngeal edema, frequently hives or pruritus and occasional vascular collapse within seconds to minutes after exposure to an offending antigen.

It is generally agreed that IgE is responsible in penicillin sensitivity. IgE is only presumed to be involved in similar reactions to a host of other drugs; extensive investigations have not been carried out. A
list of all the drugs and therapeutic agents which
have been reported to have caused anaphylaxis is too
long to enumerate in this article. Certainly, penicillin is the most common, and occurs much more frequently after intra-muscular as opposed to oral use.
Sensitivity may be so inordinate that anaphylaxis occurs even with exposure to infinitesimal quantities of
the hapten. Multiple cases of recurrent urticaria
with or without anaphylaxis have been traced to small
quantities of penicillin in milk from penicillin treated cows. Indeed even handling penicillin, such as in
mixing intravenous solutions, has led to life-threatening reactions in nurses. Urticaria that appears several
hours to days after the administration of penicillin is
usually not accompanied by other symptoms. IgE continues to be the probable responsible immunoglobulin but
the response may be modulated by antigen specific IgG
and IgM whose presence may, in fact, protect from the
more fulminant immediate reaction. Other investigators
have attributed a more direct role to these immunoglobulins. Other drugs exhibit similar clinical patterns but the immune responses simply have not been investigated. Less commonly, sulfonamides, streptomycin
and cephalosporins are responsible agents whereas chlor-
amphenicol, tetracycline and erythromycin are rarely
incriminated. Among local anesthetics, procaine seems
much more allergenic than lidocaine. Other miscellaneous medications, including insulin, hormone extracts,
transfusions and even therapeutic hyposensitizing injections, i.e. pollens and molds, have been incriminated
in urticaria.

Histamine release may produce a syndrome indistinguishable from anaphylaxis, although more commonly the
only manifestation is urticaria. Codeine, morphine,
meperidine and colymycin are commonly used drugs which
cause the liberation of histamine from tissue mast
cells without benefit of antibody. The reaction, commonly misinterpreted as allergic, is usually not as
rapid but does occur within the first one to two hours.
Organic dyes used in radio-contrast studies also re-

lease histamine and untoward reactions are attributed
to this pharmacologic property. The occurrence of occasional catastrophic events may be due to the quantity
involved and the intravenous route.

Aspirin, ubiquitous in innumerable over-the-counter
preparations, and a variety of chemically unrelated
non-steroidal anti-inflammatory compounds, i.e. indomethacin, phenybutazone, may also induce reactions indistinguishable from the anaphylactic response. In fact,
a number of deaths have been attributed to sensitivity
after aspirin challenge testing. The mechanism is unclear but it does not appear to be antibody mediated.
Sensitive patients frequently have adult onset non-
atopic bronchial asthma associated with nasal polyps;
nonetheless chronic recurrent urticaria may be the
sole manifestation. Frequently, only occasional use
perpetuates a daily reaction. In ongoing cases of
urticaria, aspirin may magnify the response in a patient
who tolerates it without incident when asymptomatic.

Serum sickness, so named because it occurred after
the administration of heterologous serum used frequently prior to mass immunization, consists of fever, joint
swelling, lymphadenopathy, occasional nephritis and an
urticarial eruption. Characteristically, it occurs
seven to fourteen days after the administration of a
drug and this variability may depend upon prior sensitization. In experimental serum sickness, the responsible immunoglobulin is antigen specific IgG; however,
definitive studies have not been carried out in humans.
Heterologous serum is not common and offending drugs
are primarily penicillin, sulfonamides, "Dilantin,"
streptomycin and propylthiouricil.

There is virtually no skin or serum test which will
offer any more insight than the clinical presentation.
In fact, the only skin test available is the major determinant, penicilloyl, and other minor determinants
mixed with a small quantity of penicillin. Skin testing has been utilized only to predict if a patient who
absolutely requires penicillin will experience anaphylaxis. Its use for other than this purpose is discouraged. Likewise, provocative tests with the suspected
drug should be performed only when it must be used for
life saving purposes.

FOODS

Foods per se, particularly grain, will occasionally precipitate "chronic" urticaria. Elimination diets are always valuable, are inexpensive, and will at least allay the patient's anxieties concerning the role of diet. Skin testing, frequently performed, is seldom helpful. For a more complete discussion of food allergy and appropriate diets, see chapter 9. Various foods, including strawberries, lobster, crayfish and mussels are direct histamine liberators without IgE involvement. Food contains a number of additives and other substances variably incriminated in urticaria. These include dyes, especially tartrazine, naturally occurring salicylates usually found in various fruits, benzoic acid perservatives, molds and/or their by-products. Appropriate diets eliminating these categories have met with varying success by some investigators, particularly in those patients with "chronic" urticaria. Acute reactions to these substances have been presumed but poorly documented with the exception of tartrazine.

INHALANTS

Seasonal allergic rhinitis and asthma secondary to pollen may be associated with diffuse urticaria. Rarely, it is the sole manifestation of pollen sensitivity. Afflicted patients experience predictable seasonal recurrences and have elevated IgE levels to the appropriate pollens. Aerosolized grains and fish occasionally produce disease in sensitized and exposed workers.

COLD URTICARIA

Hypersensitivity to cold encompasses a fascinating and diverse group of disorders, i.e. the cryopathies (Table 2). Urticaria may be an essential feature, i.e. familial urticaria, or an unusual feature, but occurs in all varieties of cryopathies except the cold agglutinin syndrome. Lesions usually occur on exposed surfaces but may be generalized and even may occur after rewarming. In some cases the association with cold is not recognized and patients with a chronic recurrent process have been labeled idiopathic until the classical seasonal (winter) pattern emerges.

TABLE 2
Cold Urticarias -- Clinical Features

| Cold Urticaria | Induction of Lesions | | Laboratory |
	Application of Cold	Environmental Cooling	
Familial		+	
Essential	+	+	50% show positive passive transfer
Cryoglobulinemia	+(dangerous)	+	Cryoglobulins in serum
Cryofibrinogenemia	+	+	Cryofibrinogen in serum
Cold Hemolysin Syndrome	+ˑ	+	IgG hemolytic antibody, positive serologic test for syphilis

     Familial cold urticaria is extremely rare, and in-
herited as an autosomal dominant trait. Characteristically, lesions occur with environmental cooling, particularly in a damp atmosphere, and are associated with
slight fever, constitutional symptoms and arthralgias.
Application of cold will not induce whealing, a prime
diagnostic feature. Onset occurs at an early age and
persists throughout life.
     Essential cold urticaria bespeaks a similar condi-
tion, but with episodes precipitated by both environmental cooling and local application of cold, without
familial basis occurring more frequently in atopics
with an onset somewhat later in life. Attacks may occur at higher temperatures with the rate of temperature
fall being more critical than the absolute temperature.
Constitutional symptoms may be prominent, particularly
if the lesions are extensive, presumably due to significant amounts of histamine release. Deaths have been
reported from laryngeal edema after immersion in cool
water. In approximately half of afflicted patients,
the sensitivity may be transferred by a thermolabile

component of serum.

Urticaria occurs in only 3-4% of cases of cryoglobulinemia, a disease almost always associated with
either lymphoma, macroglobulinemia or myeloma. Rarely
it occurs as a benign, monoclonal variant. The whealing may progress to nodular, vasculitic lesiona, occasionally ulcerating, and for this reason, cold provocative studies should not be done. Urticaria is variable
in cryofibrinogenemia, a rare cryopathy, usually occurring with carcinoma and/or thrombophlebitis.

Vigorous public health measures have made late
syphilitic manifestations very unusual. Therefore,
hemolysis, hemoglobinuria, severe constitutional symptoms, and occasionally urticaria following exposure to
cold are now rare in luetics. The features of this
syndrome resemble anaphylaxis and are due to an IgG
(Donath-Landsteinter) antibody.

INSECT STINGS, INFECTIONS AND OTHER DISEASES

Urticaria with or without vascular collapse following hymenoptera stings involves an IgE mechanism and
presumes a hypersensitivity state warranting at least
prudent avoidance, if not immunotherapy (see Chapter
14). Similar reactions have been reported secondary
to the stings of many other insects (i.e. kissing bugs,
gnats, mosquitoes). The urticaria seen following insect stings is often papular. Characteristically it
consists of grouped erythematous papules with a central
punctum which may be best seen when the lesion is com-
pressed.

The preicteric phase of hepatitis and the prodromo-
mal phase of infectious mononucleosis may be associated
with urticaria involving a presumed but, as yet, undefined immunologic mechanism. Case reports have appeared with increasing frequency of an association of
urticaria with hyperthroidism. Finally, a variable incidence has been reported in collagen vascular disease,
especially lupus erythematosus.

HEREDITARY ANGIO-EDEMA (HAE)

HAE is a rare autosomal dominant disorder. Reduced
Cl esterase inhibitor activity due to either an absence

of or a functionally inactive protein presumably leads
to recurrent unimpeded complement consumption. Recurrent gastrointestinal swelling and especially life-
threatening laryngeal edema are other prominent manifestations and, prior to its identification and treatment, afflicted patients seldom survived past 50 years
of age. Non-pruritic edema, not urticaria, is the hallmark of this syndrome.

DERMATOGRAPHISM

Dermatographic urticaria occurs in 5% of the general population and presents as the exaggerated triple
response of Lewis in which light stroking of the skin
produces erythema followed by flare and edema. It
occurs at any age and often follows emotional stress,
drugs, or infection and may persist for from several
weeks to a lifetime. The mechanism is not clear but
50% of patients demonstrate a positive passive transfer.
Pressure urticaria seems distinct from dermatographism,
is extremely rare, and develops as a result of sustain-
ed heavy pressure, generally on the hands, feet and
buttocks. Deep swelling is a major component which,
combined with the ineffectiveness of antihistamines,
suggests that other mediators besides histamine may be
responsible.

CHOLINERGIC URTICARIA

These lesions have a very characteristic clinical
appearance. They consist of 1-3 mm wheals on a large
erythematous base, are generally truncal and extremely
pruritic, and are usually precipitated by physical exercise and/or emotional stress. Hypersensitivity to
acetylcholine has been postulated as the pathogenetic
mechanism since afflicted patients have an exaggerated
response to the intradermal injection of "Mecholyl"
(methylcholine). Methylcholine is metabolized to acetylcholine. Unfortunately, the availability of this
reagent has been severely restricted in recent years
and it is rarely used in the evaluation of suspected
patients.

LIGHT URTICARIA

"Solar" urticaria results from exposure to ultra-
violet or visible light. It is an acquired disorder
and may develop at any age but it is most common during the third and fourth decade, occuring more frequently in females. Experimentally, exposure to light
is followed by extreme pruritus, erythema and edema.
Unfortunately, the physician rarely sees the initial
lesions and such patients usually present with severe
excoriations and lichenification, particularly involving sun exposed areas. For this reason, urticaria is
a clinical misnomer. In more northern climates, symptoms are generally much more prominent during the late
spring and summer months. Six classes of solar urticaria have been delineated on the basis of the specific
wave length of light necessary to produce the reaction.
Treatment consists simply of avoidance, utilizing appropriate clothing and sun screens.

HEAT URTICARIA

Heat urticaria is extremely rare; there have been
only a few case reports and these have not been extensively studied. Localized whealing occurs as a result of contact with warm materials. Testing for this
condition may be performed by application of warm (45°
C) water for five minutes.

URTICARIA PIGMENTOSA

The brown papular lesions of urticaria pigmentosa
represent collections of mast cells within the dermis.
When stroked (Darier's sign) an urticarial lesion is
produced by histamine release. When present in children, the syndrome generally disappears before adolescence. However if urticaria pigmentosa develops in
adults the prognosis is more serious. Such patients
are more likely to experience urticaria and flushing
with histamine-releasing agents, i.e. codeine (see
above).

CONTACT URTICARIA

Topical contact with many commercial materials, animal danders, saliva, drugs, pollens, grains and spices, may produce localized urticarial eruptions. Because the lesions occur 1-4 days after contact previous workers felt they represented a form of delayed hypersensitivity. More recent studies have indicated that these reactions may occur within 1-2 minutes and are therefore compatible with an IgE mechanism.

CIRCINATE URTICARIA

The "figurate" erythemas comprise a group of urticarial eruptions characterized by large arcs, whorls or circles covering the trunk or extremities. They tend to have a clear center and a trailing scale. There are four or five types of these urticarial eruptions and all have long confusing names. Erythema annulare centrifugum is the most common type with extremely large bizarre urticarial rings which may be 20-30 cm in diameter. Such syndromes occur at any age group and are most prominent on the trunk and proximal extremities. As in the other urticarias, they may result from fungal, candidal or bacterial infections. Finally there are numerous reports of underlying malignancies in these groups of diseases.

TREATMENT

Acute urticaria when co-existing with anaphylaxis requires both epinephrine and antihistamines. Those patients with giant lesions and extensive angioedema are more prone to develop prominent laryngeal involvement and bear close observation. Occasionally, the reaction consists solely of extensive wheal formation without bronchospasm or vascular collapse. Although both sympathomimetic agents and antihistamines may both effect some response, one or the other may be more useful in a particular individual. Antihistamines, particularly hydroxyzine, have a significant duration of action, nonetheless, longer acting sympathomimetics such as "Susphrine" or the time honored epinephrine in oil are preferable to frequent injections of epinephrine.

Fuller Albright once remarked that the major thorn

of endocrinologists was the treatment of the hirsute
woman. The management of chronic urticaria presents
the allergist with a similar challenge. Months of discomfort, itching and erratic sleep test the best of
dispositions; patients often become frankly hostile
and/or depressed. Some degree of relief may be a-
chieved by various drug regimens, but these should be
withheld, all emotions considered, pending discontinuance of suspected agents and appropriate elimination
diets. Simultaneous therapies are fraught with confusion and misdiagnosis. Nevertheless, in spite of a
Herculean effort, the large majority of patients with
urticaria will be classified as idiopathic.

     Classical antihistamines, i.e. ethanolamines, ethy-
lemediamines, and alkylamines are the least expensive
effective agents and are frequently used. Failure with
one class should not preclude use of another group.
The newer antihistamines (i.e. hydroxyzine ["Atarax,"
"Vistaril"], cycloheptadine ["Periactin"]) are significantly more expensive, but have been much more effective and used with increased frequency in recent
years. Hydroxyzine was initially marketed as a tran-
quilizer, but it has extremely potent antihistaminic
properties with an extremely long duration of action.
Unfortunately, treatment with this drug is complicated
by the folklore of its initial history and patients
feel they are being treated for an emotional disorder.
A combination of hydroxyzine and cimetidine, a histamine H_2 receptor antagonist, has been successful in patients resistant to hydroxyzine alone.

     Although steroids may be utilized in the urticarias
associated with known self-limited disorders, i.e. serum sickness, their use in chronic urticaria is severely discouraged. Moreover, they are usually of little
benefit. Nonetheless a small subsegment of patients
are steroid-responsive and, though unstudied, may represent those individuals with hypocomplementemia and
circulating immune complexes.

     Various unproven but anecdotally successful measures
for chronic urticaria include elixers and immunotherapy.
Immunotherapy is useful and recommended in pollen-sensi-
tive patients not adequately controlled by antihistamines and its use in hymenoptera sensitivity is discussed on pages 245–256. Non-specific immunotherapy, i.e.

not directed at specific antigens, has been utilized
by a number of allergists on an individual basis in
patients with longstanding urticaria. Such patients
may or may not have had significant reactions on skin
testing. Unfortunately there are no well controlled
clinical trials to substantiate this. It is entered
into, in part, because of the extremely benign nature
of immunotherapy, and the frustration of both physician and patient, hoping to alter in some way the pa-
patient's immune status.

REFERENCES

Champion, RH, Roberts, SOB, Carpenter, RG & Roger, JH:
    Urticaria and angioedema, Br J Dermatol 81:588,
    1969.
Harber, LC, Holloway, RM, Sheatley, VR & Baer, RL:
    Immunologic and biophysical studies in solar urti-
    caria, J Invest Dermatol 41:439, 1963.
Douglas, HMG & Bleumink, E: Familial cold urticaria,
    Arch Dermatol 110:382, 1974.
Donaldson, VH & Rosen, FS: Hereditary angioneurotic
    edema: a clinical survey, Pediatrics 37:1017, 1966.
Ishizaka, K, DeBernardo, R, Tomioka, H, Lichtenstein,
    L, & Ishizaka, T: Identification of basophil granu-
    locytes as a site of allergic histamine release, J
    Immunol 108:1000, 1972.
Moroz, LA & Rose, B: The cryopathies. In Samter, M,
    et al., editors: Immunological diseases. Boston,
    1971, Little, Brown, & Co.
Levine, MI: Chronic urticaria, J Allergy Clin Immunol,
    55:276, 1975.
Wanderer, AA, St. Pierre, J-P & Ellis, EF: Primary
    acquired cold urticaria; double blind study of treat-
    ment with cyproheptadine, chlorpheniramine, and
    placebo, Arch Dermatol 113:1375, 1977.

Stephen M. Nagy, Jr.
and Paul Cloninger

FOOD ALLERGY

INTRODUCTION

Food substances are defined as materials with caloric or nutritive value. The layman may loosen this concept and apply the word to anything ingested, which may include additives, i.e. (dyes and preservatives), bacteria, toxins and chemical contaminants, i.e. insecticides, all of which might have both allergic and non-allergic deleterious consequences. One must consider all such materials since the initial investigation of any set of symptoms begins with a consideration of all probable disorders. Indeed the spectrum of food allergy may baffle most detectives. For example, symptomotology, even anaphylaxis, may be questionable because of absence of some essential features, i.e. urticaria, bronchospasm; important events, unusual symptoms, and critical historical correlations are elusive; skin testing, though positive in immediate sensitivity and virtually worthless in "delayed" responses, borders on theatre in the vast majority undergoing evaluation; treatment remains remarkably simple--avoidance.
The next few pages are devoted to an exposition of these themes in addition to a discussion both of the major reaction patterns and the major syndromes associated with the ingestion of specific substances.

DEFINITIONS

A diagnosis of food allergy or intolerance, though often suspected by history, is based both on response to a diet eliminating the offending substance and recurrence of symptoms with subsequent rechallenge. This latter aspect is essential and rules out spontaneous and unrelated improvement. In fact, in all but life threatening sensitivity, patients are encouraged to reintroduce the offending foods at periodic inter-

vals to prove that avoidance is still necessary. Such
regimens will suffice for the vast majority of food-
sensitive patients. On the other hand, for a diagnosis
of certain types of food sensitivity, academicians demand stricter criteria. These include detection of
type, amount, and specificity of antibody, evidence
that the antibody is biologically relevant, and utilization of double-blind challenge techniques.

Thusfar, we have avoided the term "allergic" because, strictly speaking, it should be employed only in
those disorders where an immunologic basis has been
established. However, to limit this discussion to well
defined parameters eliminates a host of other syndromes,
i.e. colic in infancy, rhinorrhea in childhood, tyramine headache, in which dietary modifications produce
dramatic clinical improvement. (Table 1)

TABLE 1
Clinical Manifestations of Food Allergy or Intolerance

CHILDREN	ADULTS

1. ENT
    Rhinorrhea
    Congestion
    Serous Otitis
	1. Gastrointestinal
	    Diarrhea
	    Recurrent Cramping
	    Constipation

2. Gastrointestinal
    Colic (infancy)
    Vomiting (infancy)
    Diarrhea
	2. Skin
	    Urticaria
	    Eczema

3. Pulmonary
    Cough
    Asthma
	3. ENT
	    Rhinorrhea
	    Congestion

4. Skin
    Eczema
    Urticaria
	4. CNS
	    Headache
	
	5. Pulmonary
	    Cough
	    Asthma

CLINICAL PATTERNS

Acute reactions imply clinical manifestations occurring within seconds to minutes after food is ingested
(Table 2). Anaphylaxis represents the most serious
disorder; however, solitary asthma, urticaria, explo-

TABLE 2

Classification of Adverse Reactions to Food Based on Time Interval Between Exposure and Symptoms

Type	Symptoms	Foods Commonly Incriminated	Mechanism
Anaphylactic (within seconds-20 minutes)	Pallor, shock, pruritus, asthma, urticaria	Nuts, shell fish, beans	IgE
		Tartrazine dye	Unknown
Immediate (3 to 60 minutes)	Vomiting, diarrhea, asthma, urticaria, pruritus	Nuts, shell fish, beans, eggs, chocolate, fresh fruit and vegetables, grains fish	IgE
	Vomiting	Tartrazine dyes	Unknown
Intermediate 1-12 hours)		All foods	Psychologic
	Urticaria, asthma, nasal congestion, rhinorrhea, flaring of eczema, diarrhea, headache, cough	Nuts, shell fish, beans, eggs, chocolate, fresh fruit and vegetables, grains fish	IgE, in some un- known
	pruritus, urticaria	Tartrazine dyes	Unknown
		Strawberries, other berries, crusteaceans, shell fish, mussels	Direct histamine release
	Headache	Chocolate, tyramine- containing foods	Vasoactivity

Delayed (after 12 hours)		
Hyperkinesis, tension-fatigue syndromes, depression, psychosis, labyrinthine disorders all "allergic" manifestations.	All foods and all additives	Unknown
Malabsorption, diarrhea, steatorrhea	Wheat, milk, soy	Immunologic suspected

sive diarrhea or vomiting may be the sole complaint.
Foods with which anaphylaxis have been reported include
nuts, beans and sea-food. Other acute manifestations
without vascular collapse may result from a much larger
variety of food antigens, i.e. eggs, wheat, milk, fresh
fruit and vegetables. Although the basic elimination
diet at the end of this chapter outlines those with
which reactions are rarely reported, no food should
ever be exempted from consideration. In documented reactions, food-specific IgE should be demonstrable
either by skin tests or RAST. Unless a serial dilution
intradermal titration technique is utilized, skin tests
with normally available concentrated food antigens are
extremely dangerous in those patients who have suffered
from anaphylaxis; hence the increased use of serum assays. It has been frequently theorized that the responsible antigen may well be a small peptide produced
as a result of intestinal enzymatic degradation and
therefore not detectable with extracts of undigested
food protein. To date, with reliable assays, every
case of food allergy has associated elevated levels of
IgE antibody.

Accelerated or intermediate reactions define symptoms that occur with some delay but usually within
hours after ingestion. Typical symptoms include urticaria, flaring of eczema, nasal congestion and rhinor--
rhea, asthma, diarrhea, and headaches. An IgE mechanism involving similar foods is responsible for a significant majority of these reactions. The classification presented here may be somewhat confusing as other
authors have defined "immediate" reactions by the presence of a reaginic antibody and not by the interval
between the onset of symptoms and exposure. This may
accommodate those whose main interest is the immunologic nature of the reaction, however, it does not
aid the physician attempting to organize and categor-
ize historical events.

Reactions that occur many hours (12 hours) or days
after the ingestion of a food are not to be confused
with cell-mediated delayed hypersensitivity. A partial
list of the symptoms and syndromes reportedly attributed to this phenomenon can be found in Table 2.
Characteristically, the symptoms are highly subjective
and do not lend themselves to any form of quantitation.

Depending on the particular enthusiasm of the practitioner, the ills of the world are foisted on various
components of our daily meals. Some incriminate the
chemical contaminants (i.e. insecticides, fertilizers,
preservatives); others, the dyes and colorings; while
a last group continue to hold out for the food protein
themselves. Such theories and practices, though frankly quite popular, are somewhat lacking in scientific
evidence and depend almost totally on anecdotal support. One of these syndromes, hyperkinesis, is more
fully discussed in a later section.

The enteropathies, on the other hand, represent a
group of gastrointestinal disorders in which foods,
primarily wheat, milk and soy have been primarily
etiologic and in which symptoms are not acute but
delayed. Major manifestations include steatorrhea,
chronic diarrhea, malabsorption and bulky and foul
smelling stools. Gluten intolerance, i.e. celiac disease, is probably the commonest of these. Heiner's
syndrome, a protein-and-cell-losing enteropathy, is
secondary to an adverse reaction to pasturized milk.
Though an immunological basis for these disorders is
suspected, the actual events have not been demonstrated.

DIAGNOSIS

A careful analysis of prior allergic events, recently ingested substances and associated symptoms will
provide an accurate diagnosis in a large number of
reactions. As noted previously, skin testing may not
only be redundant, but also dangerous as would a diagnostic challenge. However, when a specific food cannot be identified, for example if the reaction were
precipitated by a salad, then testing to several dis-
cretely selected fruits and vegetables may be infor-
mative.

The alternatives to extensive food testing are specific and basic elimination diets. If carefully ex-
plained and meticulously outlined, they are much less
expensive and far more accurate. Adherence will be
maximal when the duration is reasonable, i.e. one to
two weeks, and the physician makes himself available
for the inevitable questions that arise. The diseases

involved have natural swings, and therefore rechallenge
becomes an important confirmatory procedure. Although
the physician participates in establishing a positive
response by noting the absence of urticarial lesions,
wheezing, or swollen nasal membranes, the prime arbi-
ter is the patient. In fact, continued adherence becomes a major barometer of the severity of symptoms and
the degree of sensitivity. As an aid to the practicing physician various diets are listed at the end of
this chapter. These include the basic elimination
diet, wheat elimination, milk elimination, and the
salicylate-free (tartrazine-free) diet. Finally, a
clinically recognized but poorly understood entity re-
cognizes that mold sensitive patients may note increased symptoms when ingesting fermented or mold containing goods. A list of mold containing foods is also
appended.

COMBINED FOOD AND INHALANT SENSITIVITY

The preceding discussion of acute reactions presumed a condition rapidly induced, self-limited and due
solely to a food "sensitivity." Unfortunately, a
large number of patients with elevated levels of IgE to
specific foods suffer from other atopic diseases (i.e.
asthma, exzema and allergic rhinitis). "How do you
know I am not also allergic to food?" is the frequent
and not always answerable query when wheezing or nasal
symptoms have been attributed predominantly to inhalants. In those with a totally seasonal pattern, the
response is simple. Symptoms are related to the type
and amount of offending food and, unless these are ingested seasonally, the pattern is inexplicable. One
significant exception exists. A small percentage of
patients with pollenosis suffer from a characteristic
oral pruritus and laryngeal swelling after eating melons, avocados, bananas or walnuts, probably due to
cross-reacting antigens. Clinically, many patients
experience these symptoms only during the season or at
least suffer much less intense symptoms during the
non-pollinating months. Anecdotally, other seasonally
allergic patients have noted gastrointestinal symptoms
with fresh fruits or vegetables only during their symp-

tomatic periods. This has lead to a concept termed, "the total allergic load," which implies that after antigen exposure has reached the level sufficient to produce symptoms, lower levels of exposure which normally would be without effect produce clinical symptoms. Though plausible, it has been lacking in experimental and immunological documentation. An alternative and more likely explanation presumes increased levels of pollen specific IgE antibody during the specific pollen season and cross reacting antigens. The role of foods in perennial or non-seasonally recurrent asthma and/or rhinitis is much more elusive. In fact, a clear neat distinction is seldom achieved. However, several historical generalizations may help in the clarification.

1. In children under four, asthma and rhinitis, for the large part, are due to recurrent infections and food sensitivity. Inhalant sensitivity does not become clinically apparent in most until after the age of five.

2. Infant and childhood food intolerances, presumably outgrown, may recur concomitantly at a later age with inhalant sensitivity.

3. Tartrazine sensitivity may complicate any form of inhalant sensitivity, but it should be particularly investigated in those who are aspirin sensitive, most notably in triad asthma (nasal polyps, asthma, aspirin sensitivity).

4. The concept that insidious unrecognized sensitivity to various food proteins is responsible for many poorly controlled or steroid dependent asthmatics has simply not stood the test of rigorous clinical investigations. The fact is that, in adults, the vast majority of serious clinical food sensitivities are apparent to the patient and to the physician, provided the right questions are asked.

THE SPECTRUM OF MILK INTOLERANCE

The frequency with which the practicing physician is confronted with milk associated syndromes requires a separate section be devoted to these phenomena. When all age groups are considered, it is certainly the most common, and, in children, at times, borders on epidemic. The amount of milk consumed by the American

public is considerable and, if computed on a ml/kg
(volume of milk per weight of child), the quantity im-
bibed is incredible. In addition, milk protein obtained from various sources is incorporated into various
foods such as bologna and other prepared meats, hot
dogs, creamed soups, margarines, etc. A milk elimination regimen is outlined at the end of the chapter.

Bovine milk contains the following principal protein moieties; caseins, beta-lactoglobulin, alpha-lact-
albumin and serum albumin. All are present in both
whole and skim milk, although the latter two occur in
very small amounts in skim milk. Carefully controlled
challenge studies have substantiated the etiologic
role of not only whole milk but the separate proteins.
The value of immunologic studies in assessing symptoms
or in identifying the milk allergic patient is less
sure. In 1963 a large series of documented milk allergic patients were skin tested to milk and its fractions. Although a significant proportion had positive
responses to one or more of the proteins, no correlation could be formed between these and the types of
reactions which included anaphylaxis, urticaria, rhinitis, asthma and gastrointestinal symptoms. More recently, researchers have suggested that at least anaphylaxis, immediate urticaria and asthma should be associated with detectable levels of IgE antibody; more
refined techniques and more reliable extracts may account for the discrepancy. On the other hand, for the
vast majority of more common milk induced syndromes,
(i.e. rhinorrhea, colic, cough and chest congestion,
eustachian tube dysfunction with serous otitis, and
diarrhea), the older study has not been superceded.
That is, skin testing, especially to currently available whole milk extracts, is unreliable. Indeed elimination diet remains the most effective means of diagnosis and therapy.

Milk intolerance in infancy presents a classical pattern. The normally hungry child takes the first taste
of milk then rejects the nipple; with more persuasion
he takes it again, may vomit, then may finish the
bottle; loose stools and irritability ensue; vomiting
can be much more prominent. The pattern usually sub-
sides by the sixth month but may persist for years in

milder forms as recurrent abdominal cramping and diarrhea.

"Colic" describes paroxsmal abdominal pain, presumably of intestinal origin, occurring in infants only
several months of age. The clinical pattern of abrupt
severe crying, clenched fists, flushing, a tense and
distended abdomen, often relieved with the passage of
feces or flatus is characteristic. Although it is more
common in atopics and gastrointestinal "allergy," most
especially due to milk, no single causal factor consistently explains it.

Lactase deficiency may be indistinguishable in later
childhood and especially in adults from milk intolerance. Such patients cannot hydrolyse lactose, the
major disaccharide (sugar) in milk. It remains unchanged in the intestinal lumen and its osmotic effect
produces diarrhea. Subsequent hydrolysis by intestinal bacteria produces excess quantities of lactic acid
which is quite irritating and characteristically causes a severe perianal irritation. Common symptoms include excessive flatus, loose stools and cramping abdominal pain, especially after milk or any high carbo-
hydrate load. The disease is terribly rare in infants
and for this reason is most commonly diagnosed in a-
dults. Finally a protein-and-red-cell loosing enteropathy in infants has been attributed to milk. Such
children are anemic and quite cachetic. Although
bloody diarrhea may occur, the red cell loss is usually
microscopic.

Another prototype of milk allergy in early childhood is as follows. A listless child of slightly
higher than average intelligence, is underweight and
irritable, has poor appetite, adenoidal facies, pigmentation beneath the eyes (shiners), excoriations
about the nose and upper lip from a chronic clear discharge, and a horizontal crease extends across the nose.
Often he has protrusion of the anterior upper teeth
due to chronic nasal congestion and consequent mouth
breathing. Finally sleep is erratic due to a chronic
cough and recurrent serous otitis has led to loss of
hearing. The child loves milk and drinks two glasses
with each meal. When it is suggested that milk has to
be eliminated for one to two weeks trial he cries excessively. Nevertheless, the response may be dramatic.

Obviously, the entire spectrum need not be present to
suspect a milk related problem. Solitary manifestations may occur, but the association may be less obvious. Identical symptoms occur with severe inhalant
sensitivity, but usually later in childhood. Coughing
may be a prominent and persistent symptom, but chest
is frequently clear. Asthma may be precipitated by
milk, but it is unusual for it to be the sole cause.
While whole milk is the common offender, a poor response to diet may be due to an inadequate elimination
of all foods containing milk protein, i.e. pizza, past-
ry, pudding, etc. By age seven to eight, the sensitivity seems to wane, though some would argue it represents less volume of protein per body weight. Nevertheless, adults are afflicted to a lesser degree. Commonly, the intolerance or sensitivity persists as mild
diarrhea or as a nagging rhinitis. Older patients who
have avoided milk for years complain of a characteristic increase in the amount and viscosity of nasal and
bronchial mucus after ingestion. Many adult asthmatics
avoid milk when they are symptomatic because it reduces their ability to clear secretions. These complaints, though common-place, have not been extensively
investigated.

Urticaria due to milk is very unusual and much more
commonly the result of some other food. One must always suspect an undiagnosed sensitivity to the small a-
mounts of penicillin in milk and milk products. Eczema
in infancy and early childhood has been associated
with the introduction of bovine milk, but just as commonly other foods (i.e. eggs, grains, citrus, chocolate) are incriminated when, in fact, foods are found
to be etiologic. In adult eczema there is much less
correlation with ingested substances.

Symptoms such as lethargy, listlessness, irritability, inability to concentrate, (tension-fatigue) are
common in those with other milk related disorders.
There are, however, a group of well respected academicians who have studied this problem extensively and
feel that these may be the sole manifestation of milk
intolerance.

DIETARY MIGRAINE

It must be comforting to many older patients suffering from asthma, urticaria, and migraine to read the
lay medical press. After years of being considered
psychosomatic, rational biochemical abnormalities have
been offered, and their private lives are once again
intact. Migraine, like asthma and urticaria is a final
common pathway, an abnormal response pattern which may
involve several underlying mechanisms and multiple
triggering factors. This section will not attempt to
cover the entire field of migrainous disorders, but
only that type precipitated by certain foods.

The term "classical migraine" is a clinical misnomer
because it occurs in probably no more than 20% of
cases. However, a description of the full-blown syndrome is worth-while. It is most prominent in females,
with an onset at any age; the attack is usually heralded by an aura, then a disturbance of neurological
function, i.e. scotoma, flashes of light, paresthe-
sis, slight speech difficulty and even partial blindness and hemiparasis. (vasoconstrictive phase). This
is followed by an intense, disabling, throbbing hemi-
cranial headache, (vasodilatation phase); then, severe
nausea and vomiting. Much variation occurs and any of
the three components, neurological derangement, headache, or vomiting, may be absent or occur in an altered sequence. Much more commonly the headache is not
severe enough to warrant reduction of normal activity.
Such patients without the prominent vascular component, i.e. throbbing, may be diagnosed as tension or
sinus headache and treated with tranquilizers and/or
antihistamines. Unfortunately, there are no well defined diagnostic criteria which serve to identify the
variant entity. Physicians must simply keep an open
mind when confronted with non-progressive recurrent
headache disorders.

The association of foods with migraine is not recent.
Case reports, anecdotal information, and diets, particularly incriminating chocolate, have issued from allergists since the 1930's. Nevertheless, it takes
many years for the smoke to clear. The major common
denominator in these patients is tyramine, a chemical
agent which liberates excessive norepinephrine from
nerve endings if its degradation is impeded. Mono-
amine oxidase (MAO) is responsible for tyramine meta-

olism; therefore, elevated levels may occur in those
on MAO inhibitors or with low levels of the enzyme.
In some the response may be due simply to an exception-
al vascular sensitivity. The etiologic correlation
has been clearly established in those with food-induced
headaches by feeding tyramine and placebo in a double-
blind fashion. Although chocolate does not contain
tyramine, it does contain another vasoactive monamine,
phenyl-ethylamine, which also relies on monamine oxidase for its degradation. Chocolate sensitive patients similarly challenged with chocolate versus placebo have a much higher incidence of headaches with chocolate. A list of the foods containing both tryamine
and phenylethylamine is appended at the end of this
chapter.

Fermentation apparently markedly increases the level
of tyramine in various foods. Some of the highest
levels are found in ripened cheeses, especially New
York cheddar, fermented sausage, and red wine, particularly Chianti. The concentrations in cheese are
higher close to the rind. Unripened cheese and yogurt
contain very small amounts of tyramine. Various foods
such as pickled herring, chicken liver, bananas, avocados or canned figs normally contain lower levels but
the amount markedly increases if the food is allowed to
spoil or become overripe.

HYPERKINESIS IN CHILDREN

Hyperkinesis or hyperkinetic syndrome refers to a
condition in children characterized by one or more of
the following: hyperactivity; short attention span
with poor ability to concentrate; impulsive behavior
with inability to delay gratification; almost compul-
sively disruptive; underachievement in school; refract-
oriness to disciplinary measures. Hyperkinesis is
certainly not a new disorder, but one has the impression that there has been either an absolute increase
in incidence, or recognition has improved, or we have
simply become more intolerant of any form of aberrant
behavior. Some seem genuinely afflicted with minimal
brain dysfunction. For the remainder, there are multiple hypotheses, many psychiatric, but none proved.
Whatever the cause the behavior usually abates by early

adolescence. At least, when it appears in juveniles
or adults, we label it something quite different, i.e.,
"manic," "sociopathic," "neurotic," "psychotic."

In 1973 Finegold proposed that hyperkinesis as well
as a host of other "allergic" type symptoms were caused
by naturally occurring salicylates and food additives.
Unfortunately, the hypothesis was not tested and vali-
dation was based on anecdotal material. Indeed a favorable response rate of over 40% treated with an addi-
tive free diet was reported. The National Advisory
Committee on Hyperkinesis and Food Additives question-
ed these results noting an absence of standard methods
and controls, the lack of objective measures of change,
and absence of standards for definition of the condition; in short, a dearth of currently acceptable criteria for evaluation and presentation of medical data.

In the last two years the hypothesis has been rather
well studied and in early 1977 three major studies were
reported which included a total of 51 children subjected to double-blind cross-over studies utilizing appropriately disguised diets. Only one child in this combined series consistently demonstrated the behavioral
changes when consuming food additives. Brief decreases
in attention were noted in some children receiving the
additive-containing foods suggesting a transient pharmacologic action of the food colorings. Although this
latter finding merits further study, these investigations refute the claim of global improvement in over
40% of hyperkinetic children. The preceding is not
meant to totally deter the physician from considering
dietary management. It does attempt to temper the exuberant optimism that so often fans the fires of frustration.

ELIMINATION DIETS

Diets must be entered into with cooperative, motiva-
ed patients or their parents. Proscription of foods
may be narrow or extensive, depending upon the clinical
situation and the willfulness of the individual. For
example, in a chronic condition such as urticaria or
even perennial asthma where one is simply attempting to
assess the role of any or all ingested substances, a
basic elimination diet is preferable. This allows for

the consumption of only a few designated foods and beverages. Many patients, however, particularly obese
ones, will have considerable difficulty adhering to it.
Although the amount of food is not controlled, an elimination diet is terribly monotonous and patients invariably lose a few pounds over the seven to ten days
designated as a trial. Indeed one may even want to
monitor weights to regulate adherence. Should this be
implausible, then the alternative is multiple diets
eliminating families of foods such as milk, grains,
etc. In other clinical situations, such as chronic
nasal congestion in early childhood, a milk-free diet
should be initiated first because it is the commonest
cause of the condition.

The approach thence is to place patients with suspected food allergy on a basic elimination diet (Tables
3, 5, and 9). This diet contains primarily rice, lamb
or select cooked fruits and is generally considered
non-allergeric. If the patient appears to improve on
the diet "new" foods are added. The frequency with
which new foods are added in a responding patient will
depend upon the interval between ingestion and symptoms.
Normally, one tries to add at least one new food per
day. In addition to various diets, these tables contain a list of related food groups. Finally, after a
final regimen is achieved, the diet should be supple-
mented with appropriate minerals and vitamins. This
is most important in children who require calcium
when on a milk-free regimen.

FINAL COMMENTS

Strawberries, other berries, crusteaceans, shell-
fish and mussels induce pruritus and urticaria by direct release of histamine from the mast cell without
benefit of an antigen-antibody reaction. Classically,
the reactions to strawberries and other berries occur
in children, and, for inexplicable reasons, the idiosyncrasy does not persist into adulthood. Conversely,
reactions to the seafood are much more commonly seen in
older individuals. Several drugs, i.e. codeine, appears to elicit similar reactions by the same mechanism. These have been discussed elsewhere in this volume. Indeed with the increasing number of drugs a-

vailable, changing dietary habits and food preservation
methods, it is no doubt that the old adage "one man's
food is another man's poison"is still very appropriate.

REFERENCES

Brown WR, Borthistle BK, Chen ST: Immunoglobulin E (IgE)
    and IgE-containing cells in human gastrointestinal
    fluids and tissues. Clin Exp Immunol 20:227. 1975.
Kletter, B et al: Immune responses of normal infants to
    cow milk I and II. Int Arch Allergy Appl Immunol 40:
    656-667. 1971.
Goldman, AS et al: Milk allergy. I. Oral challenge with
    milk proteins in allergic children. Pediatrics 32:
    425. 1963.
Goldman, AS et al: Milk allergy. II. Skin testing of
    allergic and normal children with purified milk pro-
    teins. Pediatrics 32:572. 1963.
Bock, SA et al: Proper use of skin tests with food ex-
    tracts in diagnosis of hypersensitivity to food in
    children. Clin Allergy 7:375. 1977.
Boat, TF et al: Hyperreactivity to cow milk in young
    children with pulmonary hemosiderosis and cor pul-
    monale secondary to nasopharyngeal obstruction. J.
    Pediatr. 87:23. 1975.
Hoffman DR, Haddad ZH: Diagnosis of IgE-mediated reac-
    tions to food antigens by radioimmunoassay. J.
    Allergy Clin Immunol. 54:165. 1974.
Ralston Purina Co. Consumers Services, St Louis, MO
    63188: Milk-free, egg-free, wheat-free, milk-egg-
    wheat-free diets.
American Dietetic Association, 620 N Michigan Ave,
    Chicago, IL 60611: Recipes.

TABLE 3
Elimination Diet
All fruits and vegetables, except lettuce, must be
cooked, or canned
Foods allowed:

Rice wafers	Beets
	Carrots
Puffed rice	Chard
Rice	Lettuce
Rice flakes	Oyster Plant
Rice Krispies	Sweet Potato
Apricots	Acetic acid vinegar (white)
Cranberries	Olive oil, Crisco, or Spry,
Peaches	any vegetable oil except
Pears	oleomargarine
	Salt
Lamb	Sugar, cane or beet
	Tapioca
	Vanilla extract - synthetic
	Water

Eat and drink only the foods listed:
Suggested Menu:

Breakfast	Dinner	Supper
Rice Krispies	Lamb chop	Lamb pattie
Rice Wafers	Sw. potato	Boiled rice
Peaches	Beets	Carrots
Apricot Juice	Rice Wafers	Lettuce with
Peach Jam	Cranberry Juice	acetic acid
Water	Pears	Peaches
		Apricot Juice

AVOID: Coffee, Tea, Coca Cola, Soft Drinks, Chewing
       Gum, All medications except those ordered by Dr.
INSTRUCTIONS:
  STAY ON BASIC DIET FOR _____ DAYS
  THEN, ON___ADD____ALL BY ITSELF, FIRST THING IN A.M.
  THEN, ON___ADD___ "   "   "   "   "   "   "
  NEXT, ON___ADD___ "   "   "   "   "   "   "
  NEXT, ON___ADD___ "   "   "   "   "   "   "
CONTINUE FOOD ADDITIONS ONE AT A TIME AT___DAY INTERVALS
KEEP A DIET DIARY AS INDICATED. ADD FOODS IN LARGE A-
MOUNTS, AND EAT THEM SEVERAL TIMES A DAY DURING ADDI-
TION PERIOD.

TABLE 4

Food Grouping

1. Apple - Apple, pear, quince
2. Aster - Lettuce, chicory, endive, escarole, artichoke, dandelion, sunflower seeds.
3. Beet - Beet, spinach, chard
4. Blueberry - Blueberry, huckleberry, cranberry
5. Cashew - Cashew, pistachio, mango
6. Chocolate - Chocolate (cocoa) and cola
7. Citrus - Orange, lemon, grapefruit, lime, tangerine, kumquat, citron.
8. Fungus - Mushroom, yeast
9. Ginger - Ginger, cardamon, tumeric
10. Gooseberry - Currant, gooseberry
11. Grains (Cereal or grass) - Wheat, corn, rice, oats, barley, rye. Also, wildrice, cane, millet sorghum, bamboo sprouts
12. Laurel - Avocado, cinnamon, bay leaves, sassafras
13. Mallow - Cottonseed and okra
14. Melon (Gourd) - Watermelon, cucumber, cantaloupe, pumpkin, squash, and other melons.
15. Mint - Mint, peppermint, spearmint, thyme, sage basil, savory, rosemary, catnip
16. Mustard - Mustard, turnip, radish, horseradish, watercress, cabbage, kraut, chinese cabbage, broccoli, cauliflower, Brussel sprouts, collards kale, kohlrabi, rutabaga
17. Myrtle - Allspice, guava, clove pimento (not pimento)
18. Onion - Onion, garlic, asparagus, chives, leeks, sarsparilla
19. Buckwheat - Buckwheat, rhubarb, garden sorrel.
20. Palm - Coconut, date
21. Parsley - Carrot, parsnip, celery, parsley, celeriac, anise, dill, fennel, angelica, celery seed, cumin, coriander, caraway
22. Pea (Legume or clover) - Peanuts, peas (green, field, blackeyed), beans (navy, lima, pinto, string, soy, etc.), licorice, acacia, tragacanth
23. Plum - Plum, cherry, peach, apricot, nectarine, almond
24. Potato - Potato, tomato, egg plant, green pep-

per, red pepper, chili pepper, paprika, cay-
enne
25. Rose - Strawberry, raspberry, blackberry, dew-
berry, loganberry, youngberry, boysenberry
26. Walnut - English walnut, black walnut, pecan,
hickory nut, butternut

TABLE 4
Mold-free Diet
Avoid the following foods containing molds

1. All cheeses including cottage cheese, sour cream, sour milk and buttermilk
2. Beer and wine
3. Cider and homemade root beer
4. Mushrooms
5. Soy sauce
6. Canned tomatoes, unless homemade
7. Pickled and smoked meats and fish including sausages, hot dogs, corned beef, pastrami, and pickled tongue
8. Vinegar and vinegar-containing foods such as mayonnaise, salad dressings, catsup, chili and shrimp sauce, pickles, pickled vegetables, green olives and sauerkraut
9. Soured breads (e.g. pumpernickel), fresh rolls, coffee cakes, and other foods made with large amounts of yeast
10. All dried and candied fruits including raisins, apricots, dates, prunes and figs
11. Melons, especially cantaloupe

TABLE 5
Tyramine-free diet for headaches

 1. Chocolate, cocoa, fava beans
 2. All ripened cheeses
 3. Avocados
 4. Bananas
 5. Canned figs
 6. Fermented sausage (i.e. bologna, salami, pepperoni, aged beef, hot dogs)
 7. Red wine, sherry
 8. Beer
 9. Chicken livers
10. Pickled herring
11. Anchovies
12. Dried fish
13. Yeast extracts

TABLE 6
Salicylate Free Diet

	Foods Allowed	Foods Not Allowed
Beverages	Milk, whole, skim or non-fat, Seven-up, vodka, coffee	Tea, Beer, alcoholic beverages soda pop, diet drinks, cider wine, Kool-aid.
Bread	White, rye, wheat or any plain bread, english muffin, Aunt Jemima Frozen Waffles	Sweet breads and raisin bread
Cereal	Puffed wheat, puffed rice, oatmeal, cream or wheat, cream or rice, and most hot cereals	All other cold cereals
Desserts	Plain Pepperidge Farm Cookies, Sara Lee Pound Cake, Homemade ice cream made with vanilla extract	Other ice cream, cookies, pies, cakes, cake mixes, gelatins
Fats	Butter, pure mayonnaise	Margarine
Fruit	Banana, pear, pineapple, watermelon, cantaloupe, dates, rhubard, figs, grape-fruit, lemons, mango, papaya	Apples, apricots, blackberries, cherries, currents, gooseberries, grapes, raisins, nectarines, oranges, peaches, plums, rasp-berries, strawberries
Juices	Pineapple, grapefruit,	All other

	cranberry, pear	
Meat, eggs, Cheese	Plain beef, lamb, veal, fish, fowl, pork, and ham. Eggs not margarine	Lunch meats, pasteurized spreads and cheeses, frankfurters
Potato or Substitute	Potato, potato chips, macaroni noodles, spaghetti, white or brown rice, wheat (kosha), corn chips	
Sweets	Sugar, pure maple syrup or pure honey, cocoa, carob, Lyle's Cane syrup, homemade fudge or peanut brittle	Jam, jelly, candy, gum, marmelade, chocolate
Vegetables	All but those not allowed	Cucumber, pickles, tomato
Miscellaneous	Salt, pepper, distilled vinegar, dry roasted nuts, herbs	Cloves, allspice, oil of winter-green, licorice, tooth powder, mint flavors, lozenges, mouthwash, per-fumes, aspirin or any medicines con-taining aspirin (Bufferin, Anacin, Excedrin, Alkaseltzer, etc.)

228

TABLE 7
Foods and Products to Avoid on Salicylate Free Diet

I. Foods

Almonds	Nectarines
Apples	Oranges
Apricots	Peaches
Blackberries	Plums or prunes
Cherries	Raspberries
Currants	*Strawberries
Gooseberries	Cucumbers and pickles
Grapes or raisins	Tomatoes

II. Flavorings (Omit artificially flavored and colored foods and drinks)
Breakfast cereals with artificial coloring and flavoring

Ice cream	Mint flavors
Oleomargarine	Oil of wintergreen
Gin and all distilled beverages	
(except vodka)	Jam or Jelly
Cake mixes	Lunch Meats (salami, bologna,
Bakery goods (except plain bread)	etc.)
Jello	Frankfurters
Gum	
Licorice	

III. Beverages

Cider and cider vinegars	Gin & all distilled
Wine & wine vinegars	drinks (except Vodka)
Kool-Aid & similar beverages	All tea
Soda pop (all soft drinks)	Beer
Diet drinks & supplements	

IV. Drugs & Miscellaneous
  1. All medicines containing aspirin, such as Buf-ferin, Anacin, Excedrin, Alka-seltzer, Empirin, Darvon compounds, etc.
  2. Perfumes
  3. Lozenges
  4. Mouthwash
  5. Toothpaste and toothpowder (a mixture or salt and soda can be used as a substitute, or Neutrogena unscented).

NOTE: Check all labels or prepared foods or drugs for artificial flavorings and coloring.

TABLE 8
Foods Permitted on Salicylate Free Diet

I.	ALL MEATS – Except those which are artifically flavored, such as hot dogs, bolgna, etc.
II.	ALL FISH – Except fish sticks
III.	EGGS
IV.	MILK AND MILK PRODUCTS
V.	BUTTER OR WILLOW RUN MARGARINE (purchase at Health Food store)
VI.	ALL VEGETABLES – Except cucumbers and tomatoes
VII.	ALL STARCHES – Such as plain bread, rice, potato, pancake mixes without coloring
VIII.	FRUIT – Grapefruit, lemons, pears, bananas, dates, limes, and figs
IX.	BEVERAGES – Coffee and Seven-up
X.	OTHERS – Pure maple syrup, all vegetable oils, distilled white vinegar, salt and pepper

May use Tylenol for fever or pain (purchase at a pharmacy).

TABLE 9
Salicylate Free Diet Plan

Breakfast	Lunch	Dinner
Pineapple juice	Canadian bacon	Lettuce salad with mayonnaise or lemon
Oatmeal	English muffin	Plain roast turkey
Toast—white/whole wheat	Butter	Buttered carrots
Butter	Carrot/celery sticks	Buttered rice
Milk	Canned pears	Bread—white/whole wheat with butter
	Milk	Fresh banana
Fresh Grapefruit		Milk
Puffed wheat	Roast beef sandwich/ lettuce/mayonnaise	
White or whole wheat toast	Hard cooked egg	Lettuce salad with mayonnaise or lemon
Butter	Canned pineapple	Plain baked ham
Milk	Seven-up	Buttered corn—mashed potato
		Bread—white/whole wheat with butter
Fresh banana	Roast turkey sandwich/ lettuce/mayonnaise	Canned pears
Hard cooked eggs	Celery/carrot sticks	Milk
Toast—white or whole wheat	Fresh grapefruit	
Butter	Milk	Lettuce salad with mayonnaise or lemon
Milk		Baked pork chops
	Baked ham sandwich on white or whole wheat/ lettuce/mayonnaise	Buttered rice—buttered green beans
Pineapple juice	Celery/carrot sticks	Canned pineapple
Oatmeal	Canned pineapple	Milk
Toast—white or whole wheat	Seven-up	
Butter		
Milk	Aunt Jemima waffles/honey	
Fresh banana		
Puffed Rice		
Hard cooked egg		

Toast—white or whole wheat
Butter
Milk

Butter
Canadian bacon
Fresh grapefruit
Milk

Plain sliced roast beef
Buttered mashed potato,
buttered asparagus
Bread—white/whole wheat
with butter
Canned pears
Milk
Lettuce salad with mayon-
naise or lemon

Lettuce salad with mayon-
naise or lemon
Plain breast of chicken
Buttered mashed potato,
buttered peas
Bread—white/whole wheat
with butter
Fresh banana
Milk

Pepperidge Farm plain cookies, fresh cantaloupe, and fresh watermelon allowed if it can be purchased.

TABLE 10
Foods allowed for cereal-free elimination diet

Tapioca	Carrots	Cane or beet sugar
White potato	Chard	Salt
Sweet potato or yam	Lettuce	Sesame oil
	Lima Beans	Soy bean oil
Soy bean potato bread	Peas	Willow Run oleomargarine
	Spinach	
Lima bean potato bread	Squash	Gelatin (Knox's), flavoring with allowed fruits and juices
	String beans	
	Tomato	
Soy bean milk		
	Apricots	Maple syrup or syrup made with cane sugar flavored with maple
Lamb	Grapefruit*	
Beef	Lemon	
Chicken, fryers, roosters, capon (no hens)	Peaches	
	Pineapple	White vinegar
	Prunes	Vanilla extract
Bacon	Pears	Lemon extract
Liver (lamb)		
		Corn-free baking powder
Artichoke		
Asparagus		Baking soda
Beets		Cream of tartar

* The canned fruits should be preserved with cane sugar and not corn sugar. Water-packed fruits may be used and sweetened with cane sugar syrup.

TABLE 11
Milk free diet

Eliminate

1. Milk, including low fat, skim, buttermilk
2. Dairy products
    a. Butter
    b. Ice cream and sherbert
    c. All cheeses
    d. Yogurt
    e. Cottage cheese
    f. Sour cream
3. Common foods that contain dairy products
    a. Puddings
    b. Custards
    c. Cream soups
    d. Breads
    e. Pastry
    f. Spaghetti
4. All foods that contain (read labels)
    a. Non-fat dry milk solids
    b. Sodium (Na) caseinate
    c. Whey
5. Chocolate, cocoa

Stephen R. Stewart
and M. Eric Gershwin

ASPIRIN HYPERSENSITIVITY

INTRODUCTION

Billions of aspirin tablets are consumed on a year-
ly basis throughout the world to treat a variety of
painful and inflammatory maladies. Physician and lay
testamonial alike proclaim its usefullness and efficacy.
Although generally regarded as inocuous, various types
of reactions to aspirin have been noted since its manufacture in 1900. Moreover confusion has developed in
regard to classifying and thus treating or preventing
these reactions. Indeed although rhinitis and asthma
are often associated with aspirin reactions, this does
not necessarily imply an allergic etiology; there appears to be a large subset of aspirin intolerant patients who have identical symptoms from non-IgE mediated reactions.
    It, therefore, becomes necessary to define reactions
pharmacologically to distinguish into which category
patient's reactions fall. Allergic reactions are
strictly defined to be IgE mediated and depend upon
previous antigenic contact resulting in elevated antigen-specific IgE, with reactions triggered by antigen-
antibody contact and resulting in mast cell release of
vasoactive amines. Idiosyncratic reactions are defined
as unusual, or individually peculiar physiologic reactions to an agent. The aspirin hypersensitivity
triad syndrome will be discussed in the context of a
constellation of clinically observed reactions presumably secondary to aspirin. Hypersensitivity will
be used to connote symptoms which are generated by aspirin which are out of proportion to those experienced
in normals. Although hypersensitivity has come to mean
an allergic mediated response in general use, this more
restrictive definition will not be adhered to for the
rest of this discussion, i. e., a patient may be hyper-

sensitive on either an idiosyncratic or allergic basis.

TABLE 1
Differentiation of Allergic vs.
Idiosyncratic Drug Reactions

History	Allergic	Idiosyncratic
Sx with 1st contact	−	+
Dose related Sx	−	+
Sx proximity	Immediate (20 min)	Variable (delayed)
Type of Sx	Anaphylaxis	Asthma
Pattern	Seasonal	Perennial
2⁰ atopic Sx	Exzema	None
Family Hx	+	−
Laboratory		
Eosinophilia	+	±
Ag specific IgE	+	−
Histamine release	+	−
Lymphocyte transformation	+	−
Challenge		
Skin test (dilute Ag)	+	−
Oral challenge	+	+

CLINICAL OBSERVATIONS

Historically, the first case of aspirin associated
laryngoedema was reported in the German literature in
1902, shortly after the first aspirin compound had been
synthesized. The first fatal reaction reported in the
English literature was noted in 1933. The incidence
of adverse reactions to aspirin depends upon the subset
of patients studied. In the general population, it is
estimated that approximately 1% of patients, if challenged with aspirin ingestion, will have one of the
above type reactions. If, on the other hand, adult
asthmatic patients are challenged with oral aspirin a
16% incidence of reactions occurs. Children seem to be
a more heterogeneous group with approximately 30% of
asthmatic children reacting to challenge.

In attempting to sort out which patients are exper-
iencing allergic versus idiosyncratic reactions to aspirin, several basic principles must be kept in mind
(Table 2). Allergic patients should not, by history,

experience reactions with the first, or priming, exposure; should experience non-dose related symptoms
with subsequent exposures; and have symptoms in close
proximity to contact with the agent. Furthermore the
primary symptoms can be asthma, rhinitis, and/or anaphylactic type reactions, which may be accompanied by
acute or chronic urticaria. The onset and pattern of
symptom development should suggest some variation in
either seasonal or contact exposure; and allergic patients often have secondary manifestations of atopy,
such as eczema, or other food or inhalant intolerance.
Family history is often positive for atopic disease.
By contrast, those patients with idiosyncratic reactions
should have symptoms with the first exposure; experience dose-related symptoms with subsequent exposures;
and experience variability or delay in the proximity of
symptoms to contact. In the case of aspirin reactions,
symptoms of asthma, rhinitis, and anaphylactic reactions
may occur, with either allergic or idiosyncratic reactions; therefore, symptoms alone may not unequivocally
sort out the etiology. Patients' whose symptoms are
induced by idiosyncratic reactions should have perennial or contact related symptoms, a negative family
history and no other secondary manifestations of atopic
disease.

TABLE 2
Clinical Features of Aspirin Hypersensitivity
Triad Patients
1. Incidence Female > Male
2. Onset > age 30
3. Onset asthma and ASA hypersensitivity within 1 year
4. Asthma primary symptom
5. Nasal polops, polypectomy, sinusitis frequent
6. Negative family atopic history
7. Negative secondary manifestations of atopy
8. Rare occurrence of asthma with urticaria
9. Rare precipitation of asthma by polypectomy or
    aspirin ingestion

LABORATORY FINDINGS

In the laboratory, eosinophilia may be demonstrated
with either category of aspirin sensitivity but elevat-

ed levels of antigen specific IgE are diagnostic for
allergic reactions. In addition, mast cell histamine
release and lymphocyte transformation in response to
exposure to a specific antigen are unique to allergic
reactions. Skin test challenges should be positive with
dilute antigen solutions in allergic patients, and negative in idiosyncratic reactors. Oral challenge may
be positive in either type, although should tend to be
immediate and non-dose related in allergic reactions,
and dose related and time variable in idiosyncratics.

CLINICAL STUDIES

     Several clinical studies have been carried out on
patients in an attempt to delineate which reactions
are occurring. Phills, in 1974, studied eight patients
with a history of anaphylaxis or angioedema in response
to ingestion of aspirin and ten patients with asthma
only. Each group was evaluated on the basis of history,
laboratory, and skin tests. Patients who had a history
of anaphylactic or angioedema-type reactions tended to
fit in the allergic group; that is, they had no symptoms
with first exposure, non-dose related symptoms with
subsequent exposures, and symptoms immediately after
challenge. Their predominant symptoms were either acute
urticaria, angioedema, or anaphylaxis, and such patients
often had a positive atopic past and family histories.
     In the laboratory they were able to demonstrate el-
evated aspirin specific IgE, positive histamine release
from mast cells in response to the aspirin antigen,
and elevated levels of eosinophils. Oral challenges
were not performed in this anaphylaxis/angioedema
group, but skin tests were positive to an aspiryl-
polylysine conjugate. By contrast, those patients who
had asthma only were found to have a history of dose-
related symptoms; variable occurrence in time after
ingestion; and their predominant symptom was asthma.
These patients had negative atopic and family histories;
negative histamine release test; inability to detect
antigen specific IgE; and negative skin test to the
aspiryl-polylysine conjugates. These groups probably
represent extremes in the spectrum of allergic vs
idiosyncratic reactions.

In patients who experience asthma in response to aspirin ingestion, there is a subset of patients who have a syndrome that includes aspirin hypersensitivity, asthma, and nasal polyposis with recurrent sinusitis, the so called triad. Several groups, including Settipane's and Samter's, have collected extensive clinical information regarding these patients. In general, these patients fall into the idiosyncratic or non-allergic group based on history, symptoms, laboratory, and skin test results. By history these patients' predominant symptom is asthma, accompanied at various times by rhinitis but generally not associated with urticaria or angioedema. Symptoms may be acute in onset and systemic in nature, thus resembling anaphylaxis. Delayed reactions are, however, more frequent.

The onset of such patients' asthma is usually within one year of the onset of aspirin sensitivity. With those patients whose primary symptom is urticaria, the onset of aspirin sensitivity is variable in relationship to their symptoms. Approximately 50-60% of patients with asthma will have polyposis, whereas polyps occur in only 12.5% of those whose primary symptom is urticaria. Patients with allergic histories may develop aspirin hypersensitivity, but with a definite change in the clinical picture from seasonal type rhinitis and asthma to perennial symptoms with progression despite avoidance of previous allergens and refractoryness to conventional management. Most of these patients are women, with the onset of their asthma after the age of 30.

MECHANISM(S) OF ASPIRIN REACTION

There has been a wide range in theories regarding the underlying mechanism(s) of reactivity in non-allergic aspirin sensitive patients. Hypotheses in the past have included kinin mediation, complement activation, directly acting bronchial constriction, and others. More recently, evidence has been presented to suggest that prostaglandin synthetase inhibition may be the underlying mechanism for production of bronchospasm. To understand the implications of this possible etiology, several aspects of pulmonary physiology need be briefly reviewed.

Bronchial smooth muscle tone is controlled by a
complex interaction of opposing mechanisms mediating
both relaxation and contraction. Present theories
suggest that the major factors in this control reside
in a balance in the nervous control via sympathetic
dilator and parasympathetic constrictor tone. It is
speculated that asthmatics have a relative increase in
parasympathetic "cholinergic" sensitivity, with the net
result being bronchoconstriction, especially when stimulated by a variety of vasoactive substances that con-
tribute additional constrictive properties to smooth
muscle such as histamine, slow-reacting substance of
anaphylaxis, kinins, and prostaglandins. This has
been referred to as the so-called "twitchy lung syndrome". Prostaglandins are locally produced long-chain
fatty acids also demonstrating a duality of control on
bronchial smooth muscle. In the lung, PGF fractions
are bronchial constrictors, while PGE fractions are
bronchial dilators. These vasoactive substances
interact with the above factors and help control
smooth muscle tone. It is well to keep in mind, however, that there are additional complex control mechanisms, and that individual sensitivity to any one of
these mechanisms may tip the scale on the side of constriction versus dilation. For example, some patients
respond to indomethacin or aspirin with a different
idiosyncratic reaction, bronchodilatation.

The prostaglandin hypothesis has been studied clinically by Szczeklik and co-workers. They began by study-
ing aspirin sensitive triad patients with asthma. They
challenged these patients orally with common analgesics
at different doses and measured peak expiratory flow.
In addition, they assayed prostaglandin synthetase
inhibition by three biological assay systems and correlated this with plasma protein binding to give a
relative *in vivo* potency of prostaglandin inhibition
and correlated this with their clinical findings. The
results are as follows. (See Table 3) Potency in
production of bronchospasm was directly related to the
estimated *in vivo* potency to inhibit prostaglandin synthetase. Although the threshold was variable, it was
consistent with regard to the relative prostaglandin
synthetase inhibitory potency. For example, extreme
aspirin sensitivity was accompanied by extreme indome-

thacin sensitivity. For each patient, indomethacin was
stronger in producing bronchoconstriction than aspirin,
which was stronger than phenylbutazone. A follow up
study using similar techniques with newer propionic
acid derivative prostaglandin inhibitors gave intermediate results.

TABLE 3
Chemicals and Drugs Causing Adverse Reactions
in ASA Sensitive Patients

Chemical	% Cross Reaction	Mechanism	Relative Potency
Indomethacin	100	PG synthetase inhibition	1400
Mefenamic acid	90	PG synthetase inhibition	640
Acetyl sali- cylic acid	100	PG synthetase inhibition	35
Ibuprofen	100	PG synthetase inhibition	15
Fenoprofen	100	PG synthetase inhibition	10
Flufenamic acid	80	PG synthetase inhibition	10
Phenylbutazone	50	PG synthetase inhibition	7
Tartrazine (FDC yellow #5)	30	Unknown	–
Sodium benzoate	30	Unknown	–

It has been suggested that such patients are particularly sensitive to histamine, and that the direct
inhibition of histamine release from lung tissues
demonstrated with aspirin is the critical alteration in
these individuals' balance mechanism. Thus it can be
theorized that aspirin sensitive triad syndrome patients have a relative hypersensitivity to prostaglandins over the beta adrenergic bronchodilating control
system, and are particularly sensitive to PGE. Aspirin
inhibits the synthesis of PGE and PGF equally, but in
these patients, due to their increased sensitivity to
PGE, reduced levels of both products lead to loss of
protection from the bronchodilating effects of PGE,
with resultant bronchial constriction.

ASPIRIN CROSS-REACTION MATERIALS

It has long been noted that there are several substances which cross react with aspirin and cause bronchoconstriction in aspirin sensitive patients. The

first and most widely studied is tartrazine. Tartrazine is a coal tar derivative with a chemical structure
very different from aspirin or Indocin. It is used in
the food industry as a coloring agent under the name
FD&C yellow #5. Various authors estimate a 30% incidence of cross over reactions in aspirin sensitive patients; the symptoms are usually the same as those produced by aspirin. Likewise, benzoates are also used in
preserving processed foods, and have a similar estimated
cross over of 30%. There are a number of benzoate-
related compounds, and patients are not necessarily
sensitive to all. In addition, acetaminophen or
Tylenol has a small but definite percent cross over.

ASPIRIN TRIAD SYNDROME

Clinically, the aspirin hypersensitivity triad
diagnosis is suspected by history. As discussed above,
the onset is usually in a female in the 30-40 year age
group with nonatopic previous histories and negative
family history. It may take years to develop the full
blown syndrome of asthma, polyps, and recurrent sinusitis. These patients usually first complain of vasomotor rhinitis with occasional characteristic profuse
rhinorrhea, thence develop nasal obstruction that is
relatively refractory to conventional antihistamine or
decongestant regimens, and subsequently complications
of infection and hyperplastic pansinusitis with air
fluid levels. Asthma is typically present before
aspirin reactivity is noted, but occasionally may be
precipitated either by polypectomy or exposure to aspirin. On physical exam, pansinusitis with or without
polyps may be noted, as well as wheezing from asthma.
Laboratory evaluation usually shows peripheral eosinophilia, especially during attacks of asthma; may show
an abnormal glucose tolerance test (not specific for
aspirin sensitive asthmatics); elevated bleeding times;
and normal total IgE. X rays show hyperplastic pansinusitis in 85-95% of patients with the fully developed symptom complex. Chest X rays are usually normal. As alluded to previously, skin tests with aspiryl-
polylysine conjugates may be positive in the urticaria/
angioedema/anaphylaxis group, but are probably not use-

ful in the asthma group. False positive results are often found when compared with oral challenge. Oral challenge has traditionally been considered extremely dangerous and contraindicted in patients with strong or unequivocal histories of systemic reactions to aspirin, and is not recommended.

Histopathologically, there are no distinguishing features between aspirin sensitive patients with nasal polyposis and allergic patients with nasal polyps. Normal mucosa is approximately 0.1 mm thick versus 7-10 mm in aspirin sensitive patients, with concomitant thickening of the basement membrane. Pseudostratified columnar epithelium is hypertrophied with loss of motile cilia. The submucosa appears edematous with infiltration of plasma cells, lymphocytes, and eosinophil. There may be intense IgE staining of nasal plasma cells, but it is not known if this is IgE produced or phagocytosed by these cells.

TREATMENT

There have been no studies to date supporting the use of elimination diets for naturally occurring salicylates in triad patients. In fact, Samter *et al* have shown that many salicylate derivatives specifically do not cross-react, especially those salicylates with long side chains. Furthermore asthma often progresses despite strict avoidance of aspirin or salicylate compounds. However, sensitivities must be individualized and in certain patients, such as those with inflammatory arthritis in whom prostaglandin-inhibiting medications are highly indicated, selective challenge tests may be performed. In those patients with symptoms of acute or chronic urticaria, angioedema, or anaphylaxis in whom an allergic basis is much more likely, salicylate-free diets may bring some symptomatic relief and a trial is warranted (Table 4). Due to the 15% occurrence of reactions in history negative patients, it is recommended that all asthmatics avoid aspirin-containing compounds. (Table 5). Tartrazine avoidance, however, imposes rigorous dietary restrictions, and it may be worthwhile to challenge an aspirin sensitive asthmatic patient in an attempt to decide how restricted the diet must be.

TABLE 4
Compounds Containing Aspirin

APC with C. and variants	Coricidin and variants
ASA with Darvon,	Midol
Percodan, Talwin	Vanquish
Bufferin	Norgesic
Anacin	Robaxisal
Alka Seltzer	Vasogesic
Excedrin	
Fiorinal	

TABLE 5
Foods Containing Naturally Occurring Salicylates

Fruits		Berries	Vegetables	Misc.
Oranges	Melons	Blackberries	Cucumbers	Almonds
Apricots	Apples	Boysenberries	Peppers	Currants
Grapefruit	Plums	Cherries	Tabasco	Raisins
Peaches	Grapes	Dewberries	Tomatoes	Wintergreen
Lemons	Prunes	Gooseberries	Potatoes	
Nectarines		Raspberries		
		Strawberries		

Salicylates Added
Root beer
Mint candy
Wintergreen candy

Treatment should be aimed at symptomatic control.
Conventional antihistamines and decongestants as well
as topical steroids may be employed for the rhinorrhea
and rhinitis with nasal obstruction. Bronchodilators
should be utilized in the normal step-wise progression,
noting that cromolyn sodium will be ineffective. Oral
steroids are often required but patients can usually be
maintained at low doses. To date there is no published
experience with the use of topical steroids in these
patients. Vigorous treatment of the secondary complications including antibiotics to control bacterial sinus
infections and the appropriate polypectomy or drainage
procedure should be performed when indicated.

Challenges should be undertaken under strictly controlled, preferrably hospital, situations with emergency
equipment available to treat anaphylactic or severe systemic reactions. Paradoxically, there are a number of
drugs containing tartrazine which may be used by pa-

tients for relief of the very symptoms which are caused
by this compound. (Table 6) Several pharmacologic
preparations, including selected antihistamines, decongestants, and bronchodilators contain FD&C yellow #5
dye and should be specifically avoided by these patients. In addition, many prepackaged foods contain
artifical coloring and preservatives and selective
avoidance is mandatory. (Table 7)

TABLE 6
Drugs Containing Tartrazine

General Use		Paradoxical
Colchicine	Seconal	Elixophyllin
Placidyl	Synthroid	Actifed
Artomid-S	Percodan	Triaminic
Inderal	Isordil	Chlorpheniramine maleate
Premarin	Ortho Novum	Cepacol mouthwash
Apresoline	Dilantin	Prednisolone
Darvon		Dimetane
		Coricidin
		Vitamins

TABLE 7
Categories of Packaged Foods Commonly
Containing Tartrazine

Cereals	Pastries
Cake mixes	Cookies
Frosting mixes	Pie fillings
Pudding mixes	Snack foods
Ice cream	(chips, crackers)
Candy	Brownie mixes
Soda pop	

Prognosis in these triad syndrome patients seems to
be no different than for other asthmatics, either of an
atopic or intrinsic nature. These patients may be somewhat difficult to manage, but aside from the relatively
rare acute systemic reaction, should not suffer undue
morbidity associated with their aspirin hypersensitivity.
Although reactions to aspirin compounds may at
first seem difficult to classify, attention to the
history, awareness of the clinical aspirin triad syndrome, and judicious use of challenge tests allows a

rational approach to both the allergic and idiosyncratic hypersensitivity reactions that occur in response
to aspirin ingestion.

REFERENCES

Farr RS: Asthma in adults: the ambulatory patient.
    Hosp Prac   113, April 1978.
Harnett JL, Spector SL, Farr RS: Aspirin idiosyncrasy:
    asthma and urticaria. In: Allergy: Principles and
    Practice. Middleton, Reed, and Ellis, ed. Ch 54:
    1002, 1978.   Includes lists of products with ASA
    and tartrazine.
Noid HE, et al: Diet plan for patients with salicylate
    induced urticaria. Arch Dermatol 109:866, 1974.
Phills JA, Perelmutter L: IgE mediated and non-IgE
    mediated allergic-type reactions to aspirin. Acta
    Allergol 29: 474, 1974.
Samter M: Intolerance to aspirin. Hosp Prac 85,
    December 1973.
Settipane GA, Pudupakkam RK: Aspirin intolerance. III.
    Subtypes, familial occurrence, and cross-reactivity
    with tartrazine. J All and Clin Immunol 56:215,
    1975.
Szczeklik, et al: Relationship of inhibition of pro-
    staglandin biosynthesis by analgesics to asthma
    attacks in aspirin-sensitive patients. Br Med J
    1:67, 1975.

Martin D. Valentine

INSECT STING HYPERSENSITIVITY: USE OF VENOMS IN DIAGNOSIS AND TREATMENT

INTRODUCTION

The bites or stings of certain insects may have an effect in man which is directly due to the toxic effects of various pharmacologically active ingredients in their salivary secretions or venoms; these include the immediate pain, redness and swelling resulting from these materials. Although it has been suggested that this might explain some reactions after stings; systemic symptoms do not occur at the time of the first exposure but require subsequent stings. The implication here is that the first exposure resulted in sensitization.

HONEYBEE SENSITIVITY

In 1925, Braun reported his experience in testing and attempted treatment of a patient sensitive to honeybee stings. He prepared an extract of bee hind parts, rich in venom-sac contents. The response of his patient to application of this extract to the patient's scarified skin included not only erythema and edema, but also systemic symptoms. Several years later in the United States, Benson and Semenov found that both venom and body extracts from honeybees were reactive on skin testing in a beekeeper. An important observation regarding this beekeeper was that he not only had systemic manifestations after stings but also had inhalant symptoms after working around the beehives where he inhaled a fair amount of bee "fluff". He had been sensitized to venom parenterally and to bee body dust by inhalation.

247

Studies some years later made it appear that many of the hymenoptera shared common antigens, particularly if antisera raised in animals were used for analysis of antigenic constituents. Because of this, and because of the difficulty in obtaining sufficient quantities of venom for testing and possible desensitization, extracts for these purposes were thus prepared from whole crushed insect bodies. At the moment of production of such preparations, they would undoubtedly be relatively potent with respect to venom, but would also be subject to very rapid degradation due to various proteolytic substances in the entire mashed bees. In any event, not many physicians were able to use preparations that were so fresh as to contain a great deal of venom, and allergists came to accept as a matter of course the observation that WBE rarely evoked a positive response in "allergic" individuals at a concentration free of non-specific irritation. Since many patients were encountered whose recent history of anaphylaxis could not be confirmed by skin-testing with WBE, it was suggested that the reactions that some of these patients had experienced might have been due to the direct toxic effects of envenomation, or possibly "idiosyncratic" susceptibility to certain of the biochemically active compounds in the venoms.

Landmark skin testing studies were done by Dr. Schwartz, and Drs. Bernton and Brown, who reported in 1965 their rather disappointing experience in evaluating the capacity of WBE to elicit positive skin tests in normal individuals. Both reports documented the extremely high rate of falsely positive reactions in persons with no history of Hymenoptera sensitivity. Hunt, using venoms of honeybee, yellow jacket, yellow hornet, bald-faced hornet and wasp reported in 1976 that in patients with relatively recent and convincing histories of systemic anaphylaxis, such histories were easily confirmed by positive skin tests. Normal individuals rarely reacted to even relatively high concentration.

Prior to our initial attempts at skin-testing with venoms, those materials were used in vitro in an application of the technique developed by Lichtenstein. Samples of the leukocyte-containing fraction obtained by dextran sedimentation of blood from Hymenoptera-allergic donors were exposed to varying concentrations of venom, and the proportion of histamine released was determined spectrofluorometrically. In this way, an approximate idea of the antigenic potency of the venom materials was gained. In general, sub-microgram concentrations of venom were easily demonstrable as sufficient to cause antigen-specific histamine release from allergic human basophils. Using their technique, it was also possible to demonstrate the specificity of each individual's sensitivity: a person allergic to yellow jacket showed no evidence of allergy to honey-bee, and the converse was also true. Limited degrees of cross-sensitization could sometimes be demonstrated between the vespid (yellow jacket, yellow hornet and bald-face hornet).

In practice, skin testing with venoms prepared either by ourselves or commercial suppliers has proven safe and reliable. Although we are not totally convinced that classical "desensitization," or transient refractioness to skin testing occurs in the period immediately following a systemic reaction, we generally delay testing until two weeks after such a reaction. Until greater experience is gained in venom skin testing, it seems prudent to use one of the epicutaneous (scratch, prick, or puncture) techniques before proceeding with intradermal tests in individuals with histories of reactions which included life-threatening manifestations. If the epicutaneous test is negative with a concentration of 0.1 microgram/ml of venom, then intracutaneous tests may safely be performed beginning with a concentration of 0.001 mcg/ml, working up to a maximum concentration of 1.0 mcg/ml. Concentrations of 10 mcg/ml or greater will clearly cause non-specific irritant reactions in a large proportion of non-allergic individuals.

Since 1975, over 500 patients have consulted us regarding possible insect sting allergy. Initially, we were faced with the situation of the beekeeper's son reported by Dr. Lichtenstein in the New England Journal of Medicine; we undertook treatment with venom provided by the patient's father after he was a demonstrated failure of therapy on whole-body extract.

The circumstances surrounding his treatment were
further complicated by the fact that his sister had
earlier died of honeybee sting anaphylaxis. We were
successful in being able to demonstrate a rise in IgG
after venom immunotherapy in this child, and he successfully passed a challenge in the hospital with a live
bee sting after his IgG approximated that of his father.
Subsequently, we treated about two dozen patients with
various types of venom, all of whom passed a sting
challenge. We then developed the idea that a controlled study of immunotherapy in insect allergy would be
appropriate.

It was difficult for us to decide whether to
compare venom treatment only to WBE, or whether to
include a placebo-treated group as well. We finally
agreed on the necessity for including a placebo group,
particularly since we had seen so many patients who had
failed to be protected by prior treatment with WBE.
This study was performed in 1976 and was reported in
the July 27, 1978 issue of The New England Journal of
Medicine. The salient aspects of the study included
the fact that it was a blind trial, that each patient
in the study had a history of some systemic manifestation after a hymenoptera sting and that we were able
to identify the culprit or culprits by direct skin
testing, which was usually confirmed by histamine
release and in some individuals by RAST testing. We
based our venom regimen on the experience gained in
the previously treated patients and attempted to match
a regimen of whole-body extract injections to the
rapid course of venom therapy. We likewise devised a
schedule for histamine-containing placebo and eventually challenged all of the venom treated patients and
a fraction of the placebo and whole-body extract
treated patients. Venom treatment was clearly superior.
At the termination of the blind, controlled aspect of
this trial, patients in the placebo- and WBE-treated
groups were switched to venom therapy. It was thus
eventually possible to treat all of the patients with
venom.

Including our initial uncontrolled experience and
the 1976 controlled study, more than 300 patients have
met our criteria for venom immunotherapy. These
criteria as noted include prior history of systemic

allergy symptoms associated with an insect sting and
a confirmatory positive skin test with one or more
venoms. We have found that positive skin tests may
persist for decades after anaphylaxis without an
obvious source of continued antigenic stimulation. It
is clear, however, that the shorter the interval
between skin testing and a sting, the more likely that
skin test will be positive. It thus appears that at
least some individuals lose their sensitivity spontaneously with the passage of time. Reisman has presented sequential studies of IgE antibodies which
support this view. True systemic reactions during
skin testing are rare; most patients who experience
symptoms when tested have transient pallor, bradycardia,
and hypotension, suggestive of a "vagal" mechanism.

The venom concentrations used for skin testing
usually range from 10^{-3} mcg/ml to 1.0 mcg/ml. An
initial scratch test at 0.1 (10^{-1}) mcg/ml is performed
in any patient whose pattern of reaction included one
of the potentially life-threatening manifestations
(signs or symptoms of hypotension, dyspnea, laryngeal
edema, stridor, bronchospasm, faintness, loss of
consciousness). If this is negative, the intracutaneous technique is used, starting at a concentration of
10^{-3} or 10^{-2} mcg/ml, working up to a maximum concentration of 1.0 mcg/ml. Since some individuals will
respond nonspecifically to skin trauma, venom skin
tests must always be compared to diluent controls.
Erythema without a wheal is considered a negative or
equivocal response, and if this occurs at the 1.0 mcg/
ml concentration, sensitivity cannot be confirmed.
Whether a small proportion of truly sensitive patients
might have a positive test using a higher concentration
of venom is moot, since concentrations over 1.0 mcg/ml
are frequently associated with non-specific irritant
responses in normal skin. It is possible that RAST
analysis of serum may be useful in this situation,
although it is not clear whether the few individuals
with a positive venom RAST who have negative skin tests
at 1.0 mcg/ml of venom are really sensitive by clinical
criteria. Thus, the physician caring for patients with
past histories of insect sting reactions must carefully
consider each case on its own merits.

We have chosen to treat individuals with insect-
sting anaphylaxis with each venom to which he is skin-
test positive. Cross-reactivity does not appear to
occur between honeybee and vespid or polistes venoms.
However, about half of patients whose history suggests
sensitivity to a single type of vespid (yellow jacket,
yellow hornet, and bald-faced hornet) exhibit positive
skin tests to two or all three members of this group,
presumably due to cross-sensitization. In such patients, treatment with a mixture of vespid venoms
appears effective. However, more data is needed
regarding the antigens in vespid venoms responsible for
cross-sensitization. Primary sensitization to polistes
is seen infrequently in the geographic area from which
our study patients have come; yet about one-half of
patients with positive skin tests to all three vespids
exhibit a positive test to polistes. We have seen too
few patients with primarily polistes sensitivity to
know whether such a history is also accompanied by a
significant incidence of cross-sensitization. Single
sensitivities are common enough, however, to warn
against the temptation to disregard skin test results
and immunize with a polyvalent mixture. The danger
inherent in immunizing with unnecessary antigens re-
sides in the fact that immunotherapy results not only
in an IgG response but also an IgE response. It is
thus quite possible to induce sensitivity where none
existed before, an obviously undesirable result.
     Our treatment regimen was designed empirically and
was at the onset based on the notion that one ought to
aim for a "maintenance" venom dose of twice the weight
contained in a single bee sting. Honeybee venom drop-
lets each weigh (when dry) about 50 mcg; thus, we chose
100 mcg as our maintenance dose. (Patients sensitive
to multiple venoms received 100 mcg of each relevant
venom for maintenance). Our choice of immunizing
regimens was also developed empirically: we attempted
to bring patients to maintenance as quickly as
possible, and found we could often do this in 6 weekly
visits. A typical regimen is seen in Table I. Our
initial doses might be 10 or 100-fold smaller than
those shown in patients who appeared unusually sensitive by skin test, but in the absence of an appreciable

local or systemic response to such small venom
quantities, 10 fold increases in dose would be made
at 30 minute intervals until a definite local response
was seen or until a dose of 10 mcg was achieved.
Subsequent increments were fractionally smaller. Using
this type of regimen, significant numbers of patients
experience very large local reactions within twenty-
four hours of treatment, sometimes calling for symptomatic treatment with aspirin, antihistamines or,
uncommonly, steroids. Mild systemic reactions are also
seen ($\sim$ 15%), most of which require minimal treatment.
It must be emphasized, however, that the physician who
uses immunotherapy to treat any sort of allergic disease must always be prepared to treat acute anaphylaxis.
    We have evaluated efficacy of therapy primarily by
challenging patients with stings from live insects.
However, we have concomitantly observed serum IgG antivenom antibody levels. Clinical protection has been
associated with a rise in IgG antibody levels against
venom antigens, but we have not been able to predict
what level might be a universally protective one. We
have thus looked for a net increase in specific IgG
during therapy. It is of interest that, as mentioned
above, IgE antivenom antibodies also increase during
venom immunotherapy, although apparently not to the
detriment of the patient. Preliminary observations
suggest that if immunotherapy is discontinued, specific
IgG decays more quickly than IgE, eventually leaving
the patient in an immunologically precarious situation.
Thus, booster immunotherapy may be necessary indefin-
itely.
    Skin tests have been repeated one year after the
inception of immunotherapy, and show no net change at
that interval, even though patients are still immune
to live sting challenge. Thus, skin test reactivity
is not useful as an index of immunity, but reflects
only the patient's persistent IgE response. IgE cannot be assessed by skin testing, unless the classical
technique for assaying blocking antibody is used (by
blocking the PK reaction in the skin of a non-sensitive
recipient.
    Of the approximately 300 patients who have been
started on venom immunotherapy at our institution,
about 280 have been challenged by a sting in the

laboratory or stung accidentally in the field but with positive identification of the culprit. Only twelve have failed to be totally protected. Each "failure" was significantly less severe than the reaction in the same patient before treatment and eleven of the twelve failures have been rechallenged successfully after revision of their treatment regimens. One patient has refused to continue therapy. Failures were usually associated with a smaller than average increase in serum IgG antibodies against venom antigens. A number of patients who have been on maintenance immunotherapy for one or two years have been successfully challenged with stings. These patients have been on monthly boosters and although their IgG antibody levels have fallen slightly from the levels present immediately after the initial course of immunotherapy, these levels still appear to be sufficient for protection of the patient. Chipps has reported that children respond equally well to venom immunotherapy; we are, however, very troubled by the possibility that patients in the pediatric age group may have to remain on venom immunotherapy for life. This raises the question of whether immunotherapy simply maintains IgG without depressing the IgE response or whether the IgE response may fall in time with continued immune stimulation.

To answer some of these questions, we currently are embarking on a study of the natural history of insect allergy in children. Those children whose reactions have been non-life threatening will be assigned to treatment of non-treatment groups randomly and skin tests and RAST tests will be followed. We hope to be able to identify individuals whose evidence of specific IgE antibody falls rapidly with time; this then would be the group from whom we could safely withhold therapy. Conversely, we expect to see the group whose IgE response persists for an inordinately long period of time; we would identify this group as the one which definitely would require immunotherapy. We then hope to be able to develop a composite profile for each of these groups, so that the criteria for immunotherapy in patients who have experienced insect sting reactions can be more closely defined.

TABLE 1

"Modified Rush" Treatment Schedule

Week	Individual Venom, Mcg. Injected
1	0.1; 0.5; 1.0
2	1.0; 5.0; 10.0
3	10; 20
4	20; 40
5	40; 60
6	100
7	100

REFERENCES

Benson RL and Semenov H: Allergy in its relation to
    bee sting. J Allergy 1: 105, 1930.
Bernton HS and Brown H: Studies on hymenoptera. I.
    Skin reactions of normal persons to honeybee (Apis
    mellifera). J Allergy 36: 315, 1965.
Braun LIB: Notes on desensitization of a patient hyper-
    sensitive to bee stings. S African Med Rec 23:
    408, 1925.
Busse WW, Reed CE, Lichtenstein LM and Reisman RE:
    Immunotherapy in bee sting anaphylaxis. Use of honey-
    bee venom. J Am Med Assoc 231: 1154, 1975.
Hunt KJ, Valentine MD, Sobotka AK and Lichtenstein LM:
    Diagnosis of allergy to stinging insects by skin
    testing with hymenoptera venoms. Ann Inter Med
    85: 56, 1976.
Lichtenstein LM, Valentine MD and Sobotka AK: A case
    for venom treatment in anaphylactic sensitivity to
    hymenoptera sting. N Eng J Med 290: 1223, 1974.
Hunt KJ, Valentine MD, Sobotka AK, et al: A controlled
    trial of immunotherapy in insect hypersensitivity.
    N Eng J Med 229: 157-161, 1978.
Reisman RE: Stinging insect allergy - Treatment
    failure. J Allergy Clin Immunol 52: 257, 1973.
Schwartz HJ: Skin sensitivity in insect allergy. J Am
    Med Assoc 194: 703, 1965.
Shulman S, Bigelson F, Lang R and Arbesman C: The
    allergic response to stinging insects: Biochemical
    and immunological studies on bee venom and other
    bee body preparations. J Immunol 96: 29, 1966.

Stephen R. Stewart
M. Eric Gershwin

FUTURE DIRECTIONS IN ALLERGY

The major thrust of this volume was directed toward
practical application of basic principles in diagnosis
and management of allergic disorders. With but a few
notable exceptions, the general approach to these areas
of problem solving has changed little over the last
twenty years. There will, undoubtedly, never be a substitute for a thorough history and physical examination
conducted by a skilled, knowledgeable and concerned
physician. Likewise, judicous application and interpretation of simple and readily available confirmatory
tests such as eosinophil smears, skin testing and spirometry remain the mainstay of the allergists armamentarium.
     This is not to minimize the contributions to the
practitioner from many fields of research in refining
our understanding of this approach. Specifically the
discovery and study of IgE and its mediators, the recognition of contributions of the major histocompatability
loci and their regulatory influences through lymphocyte
subpopulations on immune responses, and the application
of refinements in pharmaco-therapeutics, such as development of beta-2 stimulating bronchodilators, have significantly influenced our concepts of etiology and
intervention of disease. It has only been through application of studies in these and other areas of basic
science that we now have available such diagnostic advances as RAST for evaluation of antigen specific hypersensitivity, flow-volume loop pulmonary mechanics, and
immunodiffusion methods for evaluating circulating antibody reactivity to inhalant antigens in hypersensitivity
pneumonitis. Similarly, therapeutic advances have included development and utilization of locally applied
corticosteroids to minimize the disastrous long-term
side effects of oral administration; the ready availability of theophylline blood levels to optimize bronchodilator management and the soon to be realized gen-

eral use of specific venom extracts for diagnosis and
treatment of stinging insect sensitivity.

Application of currently available techniques
directed toward purification and standardization of
antigenic treatment extracts and development of more
specific therapeutic agents will be some of the immediate future payoffs. Study of such enigmatic clinical
disorders as asthma and food sensitivity will undoubtedly require not only application of these and other
currently available techniques, but the resourcefulness
and ingenuity for developing new approaches and technology. Allowing for a ten year hiatus between basic
science research and their refinement and application
to clinical practice, some of the things we might
reasonably expect to become available are more biochemical precise manipulation of antigen extracts and
development of new methods to influence IgE regulation.
Finally, and of primary importance, these new methods
must be made readily available and affordable within
the confines of the skyrocketing cost of health care
delivery. In addition, the technology must ultimately
be transferred from research benches to training programs, and then out to the community physician. This
volume has been aimed at just such a goal. It is with
eager anticipation that its contributors look forward
to realization of these vistas, and to similar pre-
sentations in the future.

SELF-ASSESSMENT EXAMINATION

Choose the best response to each question.

1. Which of the following drugs is most likely to produce severe nasal congestion?

   a. "Aldomet"
   b. Thiazides
   c. Reserpine
   d. "Catapres"

2. One of the following statements is FALSE:

   a. Anterior exam of the nose does not rule out intranasal polyps
   b. Transillumination of the sinuses is a good technique to detect maxillary fluid
   c. Clear nasal discharge is an unusual finding in chronic maxillary sinus infection
   d. Chronic cough is a frequent accompanying symptom of chronic sinus infection

3. A prime diagnostic feature of "allergic" rhinitis:

   a. Profuse clear discharge
   b. Marked sinus tenderness
   c. Very severe nasal congestion
   d. Palatal itching

4. Rhinitis secondary to milk sensitivity is best diagnosed by:

   a. Skin testing
   b. RAST for milk
   c. Elimination diet
   d. Finding of no eosinophils on nasal smear

5. The commonest side effect of intranasal "Decadron Turbinare is:

   a. Fungus infection of nose
   b. Cushingoid features
   c. Excessive burning and slight bleeding
   d. "Rebound" phenomena

6. Which of the following is an H-2 (histamine) antagonist?

   a. Diphenhydramine (Benadryl)
   b. Tripelennamine HCI (Pyribenzamine)
   c. Chlorpheniramine maleate (Chlor-trimeton)
   d. Cimetidine (Tagamet)

7. Acute antihistamine poisoning is rare even among children because of the high therapeutic index (T.I.) of antihistamines.

   a. True
   b. False

8. Antihistamine-sympathomimetic combination drugs offer no advantage over antihistamine drugs alone.

   a. True
   b. False

9. Dexamethasone sodium phosphate nasal spray (Decadron Turbinaire) is effective in 75% of patients with allergic rhinitis and can be used for many months without significant effects.

   a. True
   b. False

10. Which of the following is not a cause of nasal polyps?

    a. Dental caries
    b. Chronic nasal allergies
    c. Cystic fibrosis
    d. Aspirin allergy
    e. Chronic sinusitis

11. Which of the following is not a complication of
     nasal polyps?

     a. Increase malignacy of nasal area
     b. Infection of sinuses
     c. Anosmia
     d. Infection of surrounding bone

12. Treatment of nasal polyps may include:

     a. Antihistamines
     b. Decongestants
     c. Topical corticosteroids
     d. Antibiotics
     e. Allergy desensitization
     f. All of the above
     g. None of the above

13. The two most important pathophysiological factors
     in the development of chronic sinusitis are:

     a. Nasal polyps and rhinitis medicamentosus
     b. Nasal polyps and chronic aspirin ingestion
     c. Infection and vasomotor rhinitis
     d. Nasal polyps and infection
     e. Allergic rhinitis and asthma

14. The most effective way of eliminating nasal polyps
     is:

     a. Turbinectomy
     b. Nasal polypectomy
     c. Intranasal ethmoidectomy
     d. External ethmoidectomy
     e. Caldwell-Luc

15. Allergic polyps (A) can be differentiated from
     inflammatory polyps (B) by:

     a. (A) are pale and (B) are red
     b. (A) are relatively bloodless and (B) are
         hemorrhagic
     c. (A) are insensitive and (B) are tender to
         palpation

d. All of the above
e. None of the above

16. Chronic serous otitis media is caused by:

a. Chronic adenoiditis
b. Cleft palate
c. Nasopharyngeal carcinoma
d. Rapid changes in altitude in the presence
   of an upper respiratory infection
e. All of the above
f. None of the above

17. All of the following are very common symptoms of
    chronic serous or secretory otitis media except:

a. Mild conductive deafness
b. Severe otalgia
c. Feeling of pressure or stuffiness
d. Poor performance in school
e. Tugging at the ears

18. The most effective method of treating chronic
    secretory otitis media is:

a. Antihistamine decongestant combinations
b. Valsalva's manuever
c. Desensitization
d. Myringotomy and installation of ventilating
   tubes
e. Antibiotic therapy

19. Which of the following is a true statement
    concerning acute suppurative otitis media:

a. The stage of exudation precedes the stage of
   hyperemia
b. The stage of suppuration is always followed
   by the stage of exudation
c. The stage of resolution may be followed by
   the stage of hyperemia
d. The stage of exudation is preceded by hyperemia

    e.   All of the above.

    f.   None of the above.

20. The most important diagnostic sign or symptom in serous otitis media is:

    a.   History of poor school performance

    b.   Conductive hearing loss

    c.   The absence of tympanic membrane mobility in the absence of perforation

    d.   Recurrent otalgia

    e.   Vertigo

21. Major defense mechanisms of the lung include each of the following except:

    a.   Filtration by impaction of large particles in the peripheral bronchioles

    b.   Mucociliary secretion

    c.   Pulmonary macrophages

    d.   IgA

22. Properties of IgA which enhance the local mucosal barrier include all of the following except:

    a.   Agglutinization of bacteria

    b.   Presence in high concentration in mucous secretions

    c.   Dimeric structure coupled to secretory component

    d.   Complement activation

23. Therapeutic plasma levels of theophylline can be achieved easily in 95% of the population by:

    a.   100 mg aminophylline three times daily

    b.   250 mg theophylline four times daily

    c.   500 mg aminophylline rectal suppositories twice daily

    d.   None of the above

24. Disodium chromoglycate:

   a. May be tried as a course of therapy in most atopic asthmatics
   b. Is useful in the treatment of exercise-induced asthma
   c. Should never be used to treat an acute exacerbation
   d. All of the above

25. The usual mechanism in hypoxemia during an attack of asthma is:

   a. Diffuse defect ("alveolar-capillary block")
   b. Ventilation-perfusion abnormality
   c. True anatomical shunt due to widespread microatelectasis
   d. Alveolar hypoventilation

26. The use of spirometry to follow patients with asthma is:

   a. Of questionable value because sick patients will not give reliable data
   b. Of no value because if patient is wheezing, spirometry is bound to be abnormal
   c. Unlikely to help management because all the derived variables from the spirogram improve at the same rate
   d. Usually rewarding because symptoms and signs imperfectly reflect the degree of airway obstruction

27. A patient should be judged as having severe asthma if, on presentation with an acute attack:

   a. An elevated arterial Pco_2 is found on blood gas analysis
   b. Marked sternomastoid contraction and a paradoxical pulse are present on physical examination
   c. Use of previously effective therapy for acute attacks of asthma now bring only short-lived relief

d.   All of the above

28.   A 24 year old Caucasian man with bronchial asthma
      is well controlled with oral theophylline but
      develops the onset of acute gouty arthritis with
      hyperuricemia.   After an evaluation, allopurinol
      is prescribed.   One should:

      a.   Increase theophylline dose
      b.   Decrease theophylline dose
      c.   Continue same theophylline dose
      d.   None of the above

29.   A 10 year old girl with asthma was treated with a
      theophylline liquid preparation.   She had a 50%
      improvement of her peak flow rate on follow-up
      after 2 weeks of treatment.   Her serum theophyl-
      line level is 18.5 microgram/ml.   She still is
      feeling wheezy and dyspneic.   The next step to do
      is:

      a.   Add tranquilizer
      b.   Increase theophylline dose
      c.   Add ephedrine-like drug
      d.   None of the above

30.   The drug of choice in idiopathic chronic urticaria
      is:

      a.   Prednisone
      b.   Cycloheptidine
      c.   Propanolol
      d.   Hydroxyzine
      e.   "Librium"

31.   All of the infectious illnesses have been assoc-
      iated with urticaria except:

      a.   Hepatitis
      b.   Infectious mononucleosis
      c.   Syphilis
      d.   Coxsackie
      e.   Ascariasis

32. Which of the following are not characteristic of hereditary angioedema:

    a. Swelling associated with trauma
    b. Not sex-linked
    c. Pruritus
    d. Some episodes associated with abdominal pain

33. In which of the following are classical urticarial lesions not evident:

    a. Cold urticaria
    b. Cholinergic urticaria
    c. Light urticaria
    d. Dermatographic lesions
    e. Anaphylactic reaction

34. RAST is:

    a. A skin test for IgE
    b. A bioassay for IgE
    c. A radioimmunoassay for antigen-specific IgE
    d. All of the above
    e. None of the above

35. Which antibody is responsible for immediate type food allergy?

    a. IgG
    b. IgM
    c. IgA
    d. IgD
    e. IgE

36. Which food is rarely responsible for immediate type hypersensitivity reactions?

    a. Fish
    b. Shellfish
    c. Rice
    d. Walnut

37. Which is a leading cause of delayed type allergy symptoms?

    a. Beef
    b. Chicken
    c. Milk
    d. Citrus
    e. Tomato

38. What is the main treatment of food allergy?
    a. Antihistamines
    b. Dilution-titration
    c. Decongestants
    d. Avoidance

39. The syndrome associated with hypersensitivity to aspirin includes each of the following except:

    a. Asthma
    b. Sinusitis
    c. Nasal polyps
    d. Eczema

40. Prostaglandin synthetase inhibition has been demonstrated to correlate with the degree of aspirin sensitivity with each of the following except:

    a. Indocin
    b. Aspirin
    c. Ibuprofen
    d. Tartrazine

41. Patients with the Aspirin Sensitivity Triad syndrome usually have all of the following except:

    a. A history of symptoms associated with the first exposure to aspirin
    b. Dose-related symptoms
    c. Absence of other atopic manifestations
    d. Positive family history for atopic diseases

42. In Mendelson's syndrome (acute peptic pneumonitis), the most important pathogenetic factor is:

   a. The area of lung involved
   b. The presence of infecting organisms
   c. The pH of the aspirate
   d. The volume of the aspirate
   e. The presence of an allergic diathesis

43. Foreign body aspiration may give rise to which of the following clinical pictures:

   a. Absence of symptoms after initial coughing
   b. Atelectasis
   c. Obstructive hyperinflation
   d. Wheezing simulating asthma
   e. All of the above

44. Pulmonary complications of recurrent esophageal regurgitation may include:

   a. Chronic cough
   b. pulmonary fibrosis
   c. Severe asthma
   d. Recurrent pneumonia
   e. All of the above

45. The criteria for an allergenic plant are:

   a. It must be abundant in the area in question
   b. It must have bright, beautiful flowers
   c. The pollens must be windborne

46. What is the most important factor in the desensitization process?

   a. Frequency of injections
   b. Strength of dose
   c. Area of injection
   d. Age of patient

J. M. is a 7-year-old boy with recurrent episodes of wheezing. His attacks occur 2-3 times a year, usually during the winter months. A typical attack includes runny nose, sore throat, fever to 101-102°, coughing and wheezing. His family M.D. has treated him with antihistamines and antibiotics but they do not seem to help. His wheezing has been severe enough on one occasion to necessitate being seen in a hospital E.R. for a shot of epinephrine. He is now between attacks and has no symptoms.

47. Which of the following should be done in evaluating this patient?

   a. Serum immunoglobulin levels
   b. Inhalant skin testing
   c. Food skin testing
   d. Pulmonary function tests
   e. None of the above

48. Which medication should be used routinely during a typical attack?

   a. Antibiotics
   b. Bronchodilators
   c. Cough suppressants
   d. Gamma globulin injection

49. If hospitalization is required, which treatments should not be considered for severe wheezing?

   a. Bronchodilators
   b. Fluids
   c. Antibiotics
   d. Steroids
   e. Gamma globulin

A sixty-four year old male presents with a two month history of severe bilateral nasal congestion without significant rhinorrhea and without conjunctival itching. Mild right-sided epistaxis was noted and his physician cauterized him noting no other significant nasal abnormality. The patient has no prior history of any chronic recurrent or nasal history but his physician had just initiated "Elavil" therapy for a prolonged depression. The patient has been hyperten-

sive for the previous ten years and is taking reserpine. More recently he had developed a very mild
cough without significant sputa but with a slight
white to yellow nasal discharge. There was no fever.
Blood pressure was 125/72. Nasal turbinates are red-
dened and moderately swollen without exudate. The
remainder of the physical examination is unremarkable.

50. Which of the following would not be indicated as
    an appropriate laboratory procedure or thera-
    peutic trial at the initial evaluation?

    a. Sinus films
    b. Skin testing
    c. Discontinuance of "Elavil"
    d. Seven day trial of "Ampicillin" 250 mgs q.i.d.

51. In this case which of the following would repre-
    sent the least likely etiology?
    a. Vasomotor syndrome brought on by wife's death
    b. Rhinitis medicamentosa secondary to reserpine
    c. Rhinitis medicamentosa secondary to "Elavil"
    d. Airway obstruction secondary to cauterization

52. After the nasal symptoms have become less pro-
    minent one month later, the patient is still quite
    depressed and is not able to return to work.
    Which of the following might be considered appro-
    priate?

    a. Increasing the dose of "Elavil"
    b. Switching to another anti-depressant
    c. Discontinuing the resperpine
    d. Referral to a psychiatrist

A forty-seven year old white female had been previously in good health until three months ago when she
noted diffuse fairly large hives over her entire body.
She had only experienced hives previously as a child
secondary to strawberries. Her past medical history
was significant only for occasional cystitis. The
patient was on no regular medications except female
hormones and there was no history of any drug sensi-
tiviites. Review of systems was positive only for a
ten pound weight loss; however, she was moderately
obese and stated she had been trying to lose weight.

Her physical examination revealed a blood pressure of 120/70, pulse of 96. There were diffuse urticaria, some quite large measuring 4-5 cms over her entire body. Except for the obesity, the physical examination was unremarkable.

53. Which one of the following would represent the most appropriate initial evaluative approach?

    a. Skin testing to basic foods
    b. Complement studies
    c. A basic elimination diet
    d. Skin testing to inhalants

54. Which drug would probably be the most useful in controlling this patient's symptoms?

    a. Cimetidine
    b. "Benadryl"
    c. "Librium"
    d. Hydroxyzine
    e. Prednisone

A twenty-one year old female is seen in the emergency room for severe swelling in the right tonsillar area. There is no fever and no tenderness. The right side of the neck is also slightly swollen. Since age three the patient has experienced periodic episodes of swelling, particularly of the face and perineum, however, swelling has recently appeared in other areas. There has been no pruritus nor urticaria. Finally there has never been any significant hoarseness or abdominal pain. Her local physician has always treated her with antihistamines which have not appeared to have been of much help.

55. Which of the following would most likely be abnormal and diagnostic in the above patient?

    a. Complement levels
    b. SGOT
    c. Food skin testing
    d. C'i Esterase inhibitor
    e. All of the above
    f. None of the above

56.   The patient refuses treatment and the physician
learns four months later that the patient died unex-
pectedly. A post-mortem examination would be expected
to show:

    a.   Exsanguinating hemorrhage
    b.   Fulminate liver failure
    c.   Laryngeal edema
    d.   Pulmonary embolus

      A forty-seven year old white male has a history of
increasing cough, wheezing and chest tightness for
six to eight months. He gives no prior history of any
pulmonary difficulty and his background is totally non-
allergic, having neither experienced asthma, chronic
rhinitis or infant food problems in childhood. His
family history is also totally non-allergic. Nasal
symptoms have been prominent for the past one to two
years and have consisted of congestion and profuse
rhinorrhea which is clear on a non-seasonal basis.
The chest symptoms have progressed to a point of significant disability. His physical examination reveals
bilateral nasal polyps and moderate wheezing. The
remainder of the exam is unremarkable.

57.   Which of the following should be considered at the
      initial evaluation?

    a.   Pulmonary function studies
    b.   Sinus films
    c.   Discontinuance of all aspirin
    d.   All of the above
    e.   None of the above

58.   The patient is placed on maximally tolerated doses
      of theophylline and terbutaline. A trial of "So-
      dium Cromolyn" was without benefit. The patient
      has required periodic courses of oral steroids.
      Which drugs should be considered next for treat-
      ment of the asthma?

    a.   Maximally tolerated antihistamines
    b.   Cimetidine
    c.   Beclamethasone
    d.   "Decadron" Turbinaire
    e.   Alternate day oral steroids

59. Although the patient has not noted any relation-
    ship of his asthma with any specific foods, which
    of the following diets, if strictly adhered to,
    is most likely to prove rewarding?

    a. Total milk elimination
    b. Mold-free diet
    c. Salicylate and tartrazine free diet
    d. Gluten elimination

60. Before hyposensitization with a particular pollen
    is begun, which of the following should be consi-
    dered:

    a. Pollen antigenicity
    b. Pollen size
    c. Geographic distribution of pollen source
    d. Seasonal pattern of symptoms
    e. All of the above

61. The most important source of histamine in human
    anaphylaxis is:

    a. CNS
    b. GI tract
    c. Mast cells
    d. Eosinophils

62. Serotonin (5-HT) is directly released after Ag-
    IgE interaction.

    a. True
    b. False

63. Anaphylactic reaction to which of the following
    substances does not necessarily require IgE-Ag
    interaction?

    a. Bee venom
    b. IVP dye
    c. Penicillin
    d. Sulfanomides

64. Factors modulating the release of the mediators of
    the allergic inflammatory response include:

    a. c GMP
    b. c AMP
    c. Catecholamines
    d. Complement fragments
    e. All of the above

65. Antihistamines are the preferred treatment for the bronchospasm of anaphylaxis.

    a. True
    b. False

66. Pruritus may be a prominent symptom in all of the following except

    a. Cirrhosis
    b. Scabies
    c. Hypercalcemia
    d. Lupus erythematosus
    e. Uremia

67. The commonest side effect of beclamethasone (Vanceril) is

    a. Oral moniliasis
    b. Pulmonary aspergillosis
    c. Cushing's disease
    d. Neutropenia
    e. Recurrent herpes simplex

68. Foods with a high tyramine content include all the following except

    a. Ripened cheeses
    b. Ripe bananas
    c. Chocolate
    d. Red wine
    e. Ripe apples

69. The following symptoms are characteristically found in migraine syndromes except

    a. Photophobia
    b. Nausea
    c. Diarrhea
    d. Throbbing headaches
    e. Paresthesias

70. Asymptomatic sensitivity to foods implies all of the following except

    a. Positive skin tests to the food
    b. Positive RAST to the food
    c. Symptoms occur only with excessive amounts of the food
    d. The food should be avoided in the presence of asthma or hayfever
    e. No symptoms on casual exposure to the food

71. The initial treatment and subsequent evaluation of an acute anaphylactic reaction to peanuts may include all the following except

    a. Epinephrine
    b. Antihistamines
    c. Corticosteroids
    d. Skin testing to peanuts
    e. Medi-alert bracelet

72. All the following foods are commonly associated with acute reactions except

    a. Lamb
    b. Shrimp
    c. Peanuts
    d. Crab
    e. Eggs

73. Milk commonly contains which of the following non-nutritive compounds

    a. Tetracycline
    b. Hormones
    c. Penicillin
    d. Nitrogen fertilizers
    e. Insecticides

74. Asthma in children under the age of 4 is most commonly associated with

    a. Dust allergy
    b. Viral infections
    c. Pollen allergies
    d. Milk allergies
    e. Bacteral pneumonia

75. Identification of milk intolerence or allergy in
    infants is best achieved by

    a. Interdermal skin tests to milk
    b. Scratch tests to milk
    c. RAST
    d. Lactalbumin skin test
    e. Milk elimination
    f. Serum IgA

76. Which of the following symptoms is not commonly
    associated with milk allergy in infants.

    a. Nasal congestion
    b. Hyper-irritability
    c. Mild aversion to feeding
    d. Vomiting
    e. Poor weight gain

   A 35 year old white, female non-smoker, comes to
your office in December complaining of headaches,
fever, and recent onset of tightness in her chest.
She has also had symptoms of intermittent rhinorrhea,
and is complaining that the chlorphenaramine prescribed
several months earlier is ineffective in controlling
her symptoms. She has been taking aspirin for the
headaches. On examination, you find she is exquisitely
tender over her left maxillary sinus area, and you see
a granular polyp under her left upper turbinate covered
with a thick uncorpulent exudate. Her chest findings
include wheezing on forced expiration without signs of
consolidation.
   Lab: WBC 13,800; PMN 65; Bands P, Lymph 10; Mono
5; Eos 10; grain stain: exudate with mixed flora.

77. Immediate workup of this patient should include
    all of the following except which two features:

    a. Culture and sensitivity of nasal exudate
    b. Sinus x-ray series
    c. Oral challenge with aspirin
    d. Pulmonary function testing (spirometry)
    e. Allergy skin tests

78. Initial management would rationally include which

of the following:

a. Pseudoephedrine
b. Ampicillin
c. Discontinuance of ASA
d. Theophyllin Anhydrous
e. All of the above

The patient returns in 5 days. Her chest tightness and fever have stopped, but the headaches and nasal drainage persist. On exam, the polyp remains, but the exudate is now serous.

79. Management should now include:

a. Discontinuance of Theophyllin
b. Reinstatement of ASA for analgesia
c. Referral to a local ENT surgeon for polypectomy
d. Discontinuance of Pseudoephedrine
e. Discontinuance of Ampicillin

A 46 year old white, female smoker with longstanding sero-positive rheumatoid arthritis comes to your office after her fourth episode of severe asthma in as many months. Her medications include: ASA 13 per day, Choledyl 400 mg qid; Terbutaline 5 mg tid. During her last episode of asthma, she stopped her aspirin with incomplete resolution of wheezing, and her arthritis flared significantly. She has had 3 polypectomies in the last 3 years and complains additionally of a morning cough and foul taste in her mouth.

80. Management at this time should include which of the following:

a. Switch from ASA to Indocin 25 mg qid
b. Change Choledyl 1600 mg qd to theophyllin-anhydrous 1500 mg qd
c. Begin Prednisone 20 mg tid
d. Restart ASA at 8 tabs qd
e. Begin Prednisone at 5 mg tid

81. Which two of the following tests might be helpful in deciding upon her treatment program?

a. Skin tests with an Aspiryl-polylysil conjugate
b. Oral challenge with aspirin
c. Oral challenge with tartrazine
d. Skin tests with tartrazine
e. Serum theophyllin levels

82. You recommend the appropriate medication and she has returned with resolution of both her articular flare and wheezing, but without much effect on her sinus drainage. Recommendations should now include all but which of the following:

a. Reducing her steroids to < 10 mg in a single daily AM dosage
b. Referral for sinus drainage procedure
c. Institution of antihistamines
d. Stopping theophyllin and terbutaline

83. Major defense mechanisms of the lung include each of the following except:

a. Impaction of foreign particles such as pollen (25 μ) in peripheral airways
b. IgA
c. Reflex bronchoconstriction
d. Pulmonary macrophage activation

84. Properties of IgA which enhance the local mucosal barrier effects include which two features:

a. Bacterial and viral agglutinization
b. Complement activation
c. Coupling to secretory component
d. Long-lived memory and enhanced secondary responses

85. The following diseases are mediated (primarily) by which of the following mechanisms:

1. Atopic asthma   a. PG synthesis inhibition
2. Aspirin induced   b. IgE
   asthma   c. Ab-Ag complexes
3. Hypersensitivity   d. IgE + CMI
   pneumonitis   e. IgE + Ab-Ag complexes
4. Allergic   (CMI = cell mediated
   alveolitis   immunity)
5. Goodpasture's
   syndrome

A 55 year old female is seen with a history of springtime hay fever symptoms dating to 1952. Her symptoms disappeared in 1960 after moving from the country to a nearby city. Three years later she returned to the farming community and her allergic rhinitis recurred. Symptoms were noted to occur primarily during March through May and she was essentially free of difficulty the rest of the year. Skin test done by the prick method at a concentration of 1:20 w/v showed strongly positive reactions to all trees, grasses and weeds in the area.

86. The most likely diagnosis in this case is which of the following?

   a. Perennial non-allergic rhinitis
   b. Vasomotor rhinitis
   c. Seasonal allergic rhinitis

87. The most useful drug(s) for this patient might include:

   a. Sympathomimetic nose sprays such as Afrin on a regular basis.
   b. Dexamethasone sodium phosphate (Turbinaire) 2 sprays each nostril tid throughout the pollen season
   c. Antihistamine decongestant preparations such as Actifed given on an as needed basis
   d. An antihistamine such as Chlorpheniramine Maleate (Chlor-Trimeton) 4 mg bid to tid on a regular basis throughout the pollen season
   e. None of the above

88. Two major indications for a trial of immunotherapy in this patient might be considered:

   a. Inability to tolerate antihistamine medication because of excess sleepiness
   b. Failure of environmental control measures such as keeping the windows closed during the pollen season
   c. Increasingly severe hay fever symptoms and the development of seasonal asthma
   d. Development of rhinitis medicamentosa secondary to overdose of nose drops.

A 13 year old boy with a strong atopic history experiences urticaria and pharyngeal angioedema immediately after injection of a coricidin tablet for cold symptoms. You treat him successfully in the ER with Benadryl and epinephine injections and schedule him for a workup in your office. The following tests are available to you and are probably:

    a. positive and indicated
    b. positive, but not indicated
    c. negative and indicated
    d. negative and not indicated

89. Oral ASA challenge

90. Oral tartrazine challenge

91. Oral Tylenol challenge

92. Your recommendation, based on the results of these tests, are for this patient to avoid all ASA and tartrazine containing drugs. In addition, what three other measures are indicated?

    a. Use of topical linaments to treat muscle aches
    b. Avoidance of Screaming Yellow Zonkers
    c. Avoidance of prepackaged cake mixes
    d. Salicylate elimination diet
    e. Use of Tylenol for analgesia

93. The optimal dose of theophylline should be the dose that can achieve theophylline blood levels of

    a. 0 - 5 μgm %
    b. 10 - 20 μgm %
    c. 30 - 40 μgm %
    d. None of the above

94. The following conditions can be associated with high serum IgE

    a. Extrinsic asthma
    b. Ascariasis
    c. Multiple myeloma
    d. Exzema
    e. All of the above

95. Extensive clinical studies have demonstrated that the best source of material for hyposensitization

to stinging insects is:

a. Whole body extract
b. bee venom
c. No difference between a. and b.

96. Urticaria may be mediated by:

a. Only histamine
b. Only acetylcholine
c. Only kinins
d. Histamine or acetylcholine

97. Nonallergenic urticaria from direct histamine release may be produced by all of the following except:

a. Aspirin
b. Strawberries
c. Shrimp
d. Codeine

98. The following statements regarding chronic urticaria are accurate except:

a. Chronic urticaria lasts longer than six weeks
b. Corticosteroids should be avoided in treating chronic urticaria
c. The cause of chronic urticaria can usually be easily determined with a thorough history
d. Immune complex deposition is found in approximately 15% of biopsy specimens of chronic urticaria

99. Papular urticaria is not characterized by:

a. Involvement in young children and elderly
b. Grouped lesions
c. Secondary excoriations or infection
d. Central punctum

100. The most common physical urticaria is due to:

a. Pressure
b. Light
c. Heat
d. Cold

ANSWERS TO SELF-ASSESSMENT QUESTIONS

1.	c	35.	e	69.	c
2.	b	36.	c	70.	d
3.	d	37.	c	71.	d
4.	c	38.	d	72.	a
5.	c	39.	d	73.	c
6.	d	40.	d	74.	b
7.	b	41.	d	75.	e
8.	b	42.	c	76.	e
9.	b	43.	e	77.	c, e
10.	a	44.	e	78.	e
11.	a	45.	a,c	79.	a, c
12.	f	46.	b	80.	e
13.	d	47.	a	81.	c, e
14.	b	48.	b	82.	c
15.	d	49.	e	83.	a
16.	e	50.	b	84.	a,c
17.	b	51.	b	85.	1b, 2a, 3d, 4e, 5c
18.	d	52.	c		
19.	d	53.	c		
20.	c	54.	d	86.	c
21.	a	55.	d	87.	c
22.	d	56.	c	88.	a,c
23.	d	57.	d	89.	b
24.	d	58.	c	90.	c
25.	b	59.	c	91.	c
26.	d	60.	e	92.	b, c, d,e
27.	d	61.	c	93.	b
28.	c	62.	b	94.	e
29.	c	63.	b	95.	b
30.	d	64.	e	96.	d
31.	d	65.	b	97.	a
32.	c	66.	d	98.	c
33.	c	67.	a	99.	a
34.	c	68.	e	100.	d

Index